A Lonely Beginning . . .

I'm convinced most of the people I knew didn't really understand what I was doing at all. They looked at me as a novelty, a freak. My actual acceptance was limited. There were certain social groups in which the people were intimidated by bodybuilding and felt they should talk down to me. They tried to point out weaknesses in the sport and argued why a person shouldn't do it. I've been through these trips all my life. There's a certain kind of person who always says, "My doctor tells me lifting weights is bad for your health . . ." In the beginning, it was kind of hard for me to handle. I was young and impressionable. I knew I wanted to do it so badly nobody could stop me, least of all people I wouldn't even bother to count as friends, but many times I did question it. I wondered why I was so different, why I wanted to do something a lot of people didn't like and even made fun of.

I couldn't come up with an answer. I didn't know. It had been instinctive. I had just fallen in love with it. I loved the feeling of the gym, of working out, of having muscles all over.

—Arnold Schwarzenegger

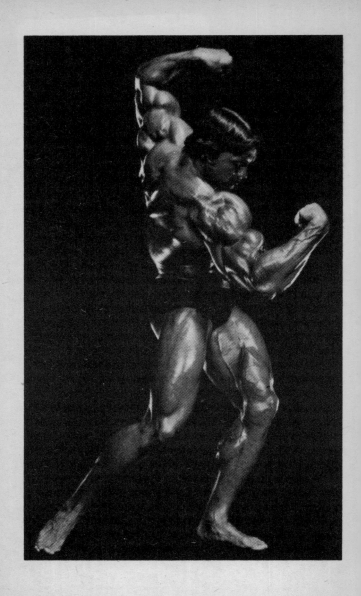

ARNOLD
The Education of a Bodybuilder

Arnold Schwarzenegger and Douglas Kent Hall

PUBLISHED BY POCKET BOOKS NEW YORK

POCKET BOOKS, a division of Simon & Schuster, Inc.
1230 Avenue of the Americas, New York, N.Y. 10020

Photo Credits

To My Mother

To Charles Gaines and George Butler, whose genuine enthusiasm, energy and talent changed the sport of bodybuilding and who I am honored to count among my closest friends.

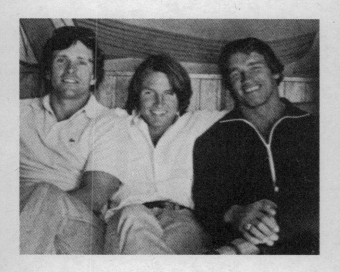

TITLES WON

1965 Jr. Mr. Europe (Germany)
1966 Best Built Man of Europe (Germany)
1966 Mr. Europe (Germany)
1966 International Powerlifting Championship (Germany)
1967 NABBA Mr. Universe, amateur (London)
1968 NABBA Mr. Universe, professional (London)
1968 German Powerlifting Championship
1968 IFBB Mr. International (Mexico)
1969 IFBB Mr. Universe, amateur (New York)
1969 NABBA Mr. Universe, professional (London)
1970 NABBA Mr. Universe, professional (London)
1970 Mr. World (Columbus, Ohio)
1970 IFBB Mr. Olympia (New York)
1971 IFBB Mr. Olympia (Paris)
1972 IFBB Mr. Olympia (Essen, Germany)
1973 IFBB Mr. Olympia (New York)
1974 IFBB Mr. Olympia (New York)
1975 IFBB Mr. Olympia (Pretoria, South Africa)

PART ONE

Chapter One

"Arnold! Arnold!"

I can still hear them, the voices of my friends, the lifeguards, bodybuilders, the weight lifters, booming up from the lake where they were working out in the grass and trees.

"Arnold—come on!" cried Karl, the young doctor who had become my friend at the gym . . .

It was the summer I turned fifteen, a magical season for me because that year I'd discovered exactly what I wanted to do with my life. It was more than a young boy's mere pipe dream of a distant, hazy future—confused fantasies of being a fireman, detective, sailor, test pilot, or spy. I *knew* I was going to be a bodybuilder. It wasn't simply that either. I would be the best bodybuilder in the world, the greatest, the best-built man.

I'm not exactly sure why I chose bodybuilding, except that I loved it. I loved it from the first moment my fingers closed around a barbell and I felt the challenge and exhilaration of hoisting the heavy steel plates above my head.

I had always been involved in sports through my father, a tall, sturdy man who was himself a champion at ice curling. We were a physical family, oriented toward training, good eating, and keeping the body fit and healthy. With my father's encouragement, I first got into organized competitive sports when I was ten. I joined a soccer team that even had uniforms and a regular three-days-a-week training schedule. I threw myself into it and played soccer passionately for almost five years.

However, by the time I was thirteen team sports no longer satisfied me. I was already off on an individual trip. I disliked it when we won a game and I didn't get personal recognition. The only time I really felt rewarded was when I was singled out as being best. I decided to try some individual sports. I ran, I swam, I boxed; I got into competition, throwing javelin and shot put. Although I did well with them, none of those things felt right to me. Then our coach decided that lifting weights for an hour once a week would be a good way to condition us for playing soccer.

I still remember that first visit to the bodybuilding gym. I had never seen anyone lifting weights before. Those guys were huge and brutal. I found myself walking around them, staring at muscles I couldn't even name, muscles I'd never even seen before. The weight lifters shone with sweat; they were powerful looking, Herculean. And there it was before me—my life, the answer I'd been seeking. It clicked. It was something I suddenly just seemed to reach out and find, as if I'd been crossing a suspended bridge and finally stepped off onto solid ground.

I started lifting weights just for my legs, which was what we needed most for playing soccer. The bodybuilders noticed immediately how hard I was working out. Considering my age, fifteen, I was squatting with some pretty heavy weight. They encouraged me to go into bodybuilding. I was 6 feet tall and slender, weighing only 150 pounds; but I did have a good athletic physique and my muscles responded surprisingly fast under training. I think those guys saw that. Because of my build I'd always had it easier at sports than most boys my age. But I had it tougher than a lot of my teammates and companions because I wanted more, I demanded more of myself

That summer the bodybuilders took me on as their protégé. They put me through a series of exercises, which we did together beside a lake near Graz, my hometown in Austria. It was a program they used simply to stay limber. We worked without weights. We did chin-ups on the branches of trees. We held each other's legs and did handstand push-ups. Leg raises, sit-ups, twists, and squats were all included in a simple routine to get our bodies tuned and ready for the gym.

It wasn't until the end of the summer that I got into real weight training. Once I started, though, it didn't take long. After two or three months with the bodybuilders, I was literally addicted. The guys I hung out with were all much older. Karl Gerstl, the doctor, was twenty-eight, Kurt Manul thirty-two, and Helmut Knaur was fifty. Each of them became a father image for me. I listened less to my own father. These weight lifters were my new heroes. I was in awe of them, of their size, of the control they had over their bodies.

I was introduced to actual weight training through a tough basic program put together by these bodybuilders. The one hour a week we had trained for soccer was no longer enough to satisfy my craving for working out. I signed up to go to the gym three times a week. I loved the feel of the cold iron and steel warming to my touch and the sounds and smells of the gym. And I still love it. There is nothing I would sooner hear than the sound of heavy steel plates ringing as they are threaded onto the bar or dropped back to the rack after a strenuous lift.

I remember the first real workout I had as vividly as if it were last night. I rode my bike to the gym, which was eight miles from the village where I lived. I used barbells, dumbbells and machines. The guys warned me that I'd get sore, but it didn't seem to be having any effect. I thought I must be beyond that. Then, after the workout, I started riding home and fell off my bike. I was so weak I couldn't make my hands hold on. I had

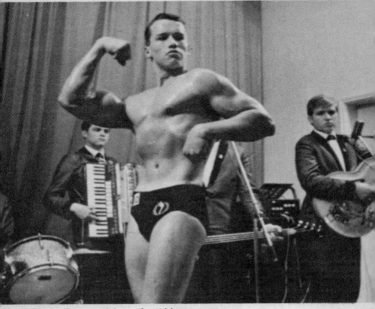

Me at sixteen, doing a front biceps pose

no feeling in my legs: they were noodles. I was numb, my whole body buzzing. I pushed the bike for a while, leaning on it. Half a mile farther, I tried to ride it again, fell off again, and then just pushed it the rest of the way home. This was my first experience with weight training, and I was crazy for it.

The next morning I couldn't even lift my arm to comb my hair. Each time I tried, pain shot through every muscle in my shoulder and arm. I couldn't hold the comb. I tried to drink coffee and spilled it all over the table. I was helpless.

"What's wrong, Arnold?" my mother asked. She came over from the stove and peered at me. "What is it?" She bent down to look closer as she mopped up the spilled coffee.

"I'm just sore," I told her. "My muscles are stiff."

"Look at this boy!" she called out to my father. "Look what he's doing to himself."

My father came in, doing up his tie. He was always neat, his hair slicked back smooth, his mustache trimmed to a line. He laughed and said I'd limber up.

But my mother kept on. "Why, Arnold? Why do you want to do it to yourself?"

I couldn't be bothered with what my mother felt. Seeing new changes in my body, feeling them, turned me on. It was the first time I'd ever felt every one of my muscles. It was the first time those sensations had registered in my mind, the first time my mind knew my thighs, calves and forearms were more than just limbs. I felt the muscles in my triceps aching, and I knew why they were called triceps—because there are three muscles in there. They were all registered in my mind, written there with sharp little jabs of pain. I learned that this pain meant progress. Each time my muscles were sore from a workout, I knew they were growing.

I could not have chosen a less popular sport. My school friends thought I was crazy. But I didn't care. My only thoughts were of going ahead, building muscles and more muscles. I had almost no time to relax and think about bodybuilding in any other terms. I remember certain people trying to put negative thoughts into my mind, trying to persuade me to slow down. But I had found the thing to which I wanted to devote my total energies and there was no stopping me. My drive was unusual, I talked differently than my friends; I was hungrier for success than anyone I knew.

I started to live for being in the gym. I had a new language—reps, sets, forced reps, presses. I had resisted memorizing anatomy in school; now I was eager to know it. Around the gym my new friends spoke of biceps, triceps, latissimus dorsi, trapezius, obliques. I

spent hours going through the American magazines
Muscle Builder and *Mr. America*. Karl, the doctor,
knew English and I had him translating anytime he was
free. I saw my first photographs of Muscle Beach; I
saw Larry Scott, Ray Routledge, and Serge Nubret.
The magazines were full of success stories. The advantages of having a well-developed body were incompar-
able. Guys like Doug Stroll and Steve Reeves were in
the movies because they had worked out and created
great physiques.

In one of those magazines I saw my first photograph
of Reg Park. He was on a page facing Jack Delinger. I
responded immediately to Reg Park's rough, massive
look. The man was an animal. That's the way I wanted
to be—ultimately: big. I wanted to be a big guy. I
didn't want to be delicate. I dreamed of big deltoids,
big pecs, big thighs, big calves; I wanted every muscle
to explode and be huge. I dreamed about being gigantic. Reg Park was the epitome of that dream, the biggest, most powerful person in bodybuilding.

From then on in my mid-teens, I kept my batteries
charged with the adventure movies of Steve Reeves,
Mark Forrest, Brad Harris, Gordon Mitchell, and Reg
Park. I admired Reg Park more than the others. He
was rugged, everything I thought a man should be. I
recall seeing him for the first time on the screen. The
film was *Hercules and the Vampires,* a picture in
which the hero had to rid the earth of an invasion of
thousands of bloodthirsty vampires. Reg Park looked
so magnificent in the role of Hercules I was transfixed.
And, sitting there in the theater, I knew that was going
to be me. I would look like Reg Park. I studied every
move he made, every gesture. . . . Suddenly I realized
the house lights were on and everyone else had walked
out.

From that point on, my life was utterly dominated
by Reg Park. His image was my ideal. It was fixed
indelibly in my mind. All my friends were more impressed by Steve Reeves, but I didn't like him. Reg

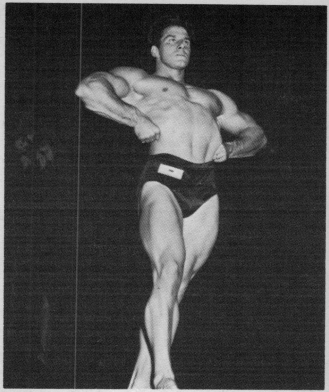

Reg Park

Park had more of a rough look, a powerful look, while
Steve Reeves seemed elegant, smooth, polished. I
knew in my mind that I was not geared for elegance. I
wanted to be massive. It was the difference between
cologne and sweat.

I found out everything I could about Reg Park. I
bought all the magazines that published his programs.
I learned how he started training, what he ate, how he
lived, and how he did his workouts. I became obsessed

with Reg Park; he was the image in front of me from the time I started training. The more I focused in on this image and worked and grew, the more I saw it was real and possible for me to be like him. Even Karl and Kurt could see it. They predicted that it would happen within five years.

But I didn't think I could wait five years. I had this insatiable drive to get there sooner. Whereas most people were satisfied to train two or three times a week, I quickly escalated my program to six workouts a week.

My father was baffled by my eagerness. "Don't do it, Arnold," he said. "You'll overtrain, you'll over-work yourself."

"I'm all right," I said. "I'm doing it gradually."

"Yes," he said. "But what will you do with all these muscles once you've got them?"

"I want to be the best-built man in the world," I said frankly.

That made him sigh and shake his head.

"Then I want to go to America and be in movies. I want to be an actor."

"America?"

"Yes—America."

"My god!" he cried. He went into the kitchen and told my mother, "I think we better go to the doctor with this one, he's sick in the head."

He was genuinely worried about me. He felt I wasn't normal. And of course he was right. With my desire and my drive, I definitely wasn't normal. Normal people can be happy with a regular life. I was different. I felt there was more to life than just plodding through an average existence. I'd always been impressed by stories of greatness and power. Caesar, Charlemagne, Napoleon were names I knew and re-membered. I wanted to do something special, to be recognized as the best. I saw bodybuilding as the vehi-cle that would take me to the top, and I put all my energy into it.

Six days a week, I trained, constantly working to increase the amount of weight I could handle and the length of time I could stay in the gym. I had this fixed idea of building a body like Reg Park's. The model was there in my mind; I only had to grow enough to fill it. My dreams went beyond a spectacular body. Once I had that, I knew what it would do for me. I'd get into the movies and build gymnasiums all over the world. I'd create an empire.

Reg Park became my father image. I pasted his pictures on all the walls of my bedroom. I read everything about him that was printed in German; I had Karl translate the English stories for me. I studied every photograph of him I could get my hands on—noting the size of his chest, arms, thighs, back and abdominals. This inspired me to work even harder. When I felt my lungs burning as though they would burst and my veins bulging with blood, I loved it. I knew then that I was growing, making one more step toward becoming like Reg Park. I wanted that body and I didn't care what I had to go through to get it.

That winter my father informed me I could only go to the gym three times a week—he didn't want me away from home every evening. To get around his curfew, I put together a gymnasium at home.

The house we lived in was three hundred years old. It had been built originally by part of the Royal family. Upon moving out years before, they had stipulated that two people should inhabit the house: the Chief of Police for the area around Graz, a position my father held at that time, and the ranger in charge of all forests in the vicinity. For a hundred years it had been the custom for these two people to stay there. Our family lived upstairs and the forest ranger had the downstairs.

The house was built like a castle. The floors were solid and the walls were about five feet thick. It was a good place to have a gymnasium. The walls and floor could take the punishment of heavy weight. I had the basic equipment, such as benches and simple machines, designed and welded for me. My weight room was not heated, so naturally in cold weather it was freezing. I didn't care. I trained without heat, even on days when the temperature went below zero.

Three nights a week I went to the gym in town. I either had to walk or ride my bike eight miles home after ten o'clock. I didn't really mind the eight miles. I knew it was helping my body, increasing the strength of my legs and lungs.

The only real problem I had with training at home was to get someone to work out with me. Already, since my experiences at the lake, I was a strong believer in training partners. I needed someone not only to teach me but to inspire me. I trained better, harder, if I was around someone whose enthusiasm was as strong as mine and who would be impressed by my enthusiasm. That first winter, I trained with Karl Gerstl, the doctor who had helped me with my initial program. Aside from his usefulness as a translator, it was especially helpful to be around Karl. He knew everything about the body. He was serious and worked hard. We trained the same way, except our goals and our diets were different: I wanted to gain weight, to bulk up; Karl wanted to lose it. But Karl gave me the boost I needed.

There were certain days when something held me back and I didn't train as hard as on other days. That was inexplicable to me. Some days nothing could hold me back. Other days I'd be down. On the down days I couldn't handle anywhere near my normal amount of weight. It puzzled me. Karl and I discussed it. He had read a great deal of psychology (at fifteen I barely knew the word, though his argument made good sense and in fact helped lay the foundation for my later thinking). "It's not your body, Arnold. Your body can't change that much from one day to the next. It's in your mind. On some days your goals are just clearer. On the bad days you need someone to help get

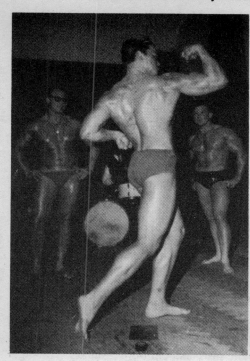

A rear view of
me at sixteen

you going. It's like when you ride a bicycle behind a
bus and get caught up in the slipstream. The wind
sucks you along with it. You just need some prodding,
some challenge."

Karl was right. Every month, I had at least a week
when I didn't really want to train and I questioned
myself: Why should I train hard if I don't feel like it?
These were the days Karl pulled me out of it. He'd
say, "Man, I feel great today! I want to do bench presses. Let's do twenty-five instead of twenty. How
about a contest? Ten shillings to the one who does the
most bench presses."

It worked perfectly. He forced me to get off my butt, to get my sluggish body moving. It became extremely important to have somebody standing behind me saying, "Let's do more, Arnold. Come on—another set, one more rep." And it was just as important for me to help somebody else. Watching him work out, encouraging him, somehow drove me on to do an even tougher set.

I discovered that the secret of successful workouts had to do with competition. For me there was never any monkey business. I wanted to compete in bodybuilding. The small competitions with Karl took me from day to day. But my first goal was to win Mr. Austria (in the end, I never even entered the contest— by then circumstances had already taken me beyond it). This initial goal inspired me to increase my program and steadily work harder. My training sessions stretched out to two hours a day. I kept adding weight, increasing the number of reps, bombing my muscles furiously.

From the beginning, I was a believer in the basic movements, because that was Reg Park's preference. At the times Reg hadn't accelerated his workouts for some major competition, he would stay with the basic exercises—bench presses, chin-ups, squats, rowing, barbell curls, wrist curls, pullovers, leg extensions, calf raises. These were the movements that worked most directly on all the body parts. I was following his example to the letter. And as it turned out, I could hardly have chosen more wisely. The basic exercises were creating for me a rugged foundation, a core of muscle I could later build upon for a winning body. Reg Park's theory was that first you have to build the mass and then chisel it down to get the quality; you work on your body the way a sculptor would work on a piece of clay or wood or steel. You rough it out—the more carefully, the more thoroughly, the better—then you start to cut and define. You work it down gradually until it's ready to be rubbed and polished. And that's when you really know about the foundation. Then all the faults of poor early training stand out as hopeless, almost irreparable flaws.

I was building up, bulking, going after the mass, which to me meant 250 pounds of sheer body weight. At that time, I didn't care about my waist or anything else that would give me a symmetrical look. I just wanted to build a gigantic 250-pound body by handling a lot of weight and blasting my muscles. My mind was into looking huge, into being awesome and powerful. I saw it working. My muscles began bursting out all over. And I knew I was on my way.

Chapter Two

Before long, people began looking at me as a special person. Partly this was the result of my own changing attitude about myself. I was growing, getting bigger, gaining confidence. I was given consideration I had never received before; it was as though I were the son of a millionaire. I'd walk into a room at school and my classmates would offer me food or ask if they could help me with my homework. Even my teachers treated me differently. Especially after I started winning trophies in the weight-lifting contests I entered.

This strange new attitude toward me had an incredible effect on my ego. It supplied me with something I had been craving. I'm not sure why I had this need for special attention. Perhaps it was because I had an older brother who'd received more than his share of attention from our father. Whatever the reason, I had a strong desire to be noticed, to be praised. I basked in this new flood of attention. I turned even negative responses to my own satisfaction.

I'm convinced most of the people I knew didn't really understand what I was doing at all. They looked at me as a novelty, a freak. My actual acceptance was limited. There were certain social groups in which the people were intimidated by bodybuilding and felt they should talk down to me. They tried to point out weaknesses in the sport and argued why a person shouldn't do it. I've been through these trips all my life. There's a certain kind of person who always says, "My doctor tells me lifting weights is bad for your health. . . ." In the beginning, it was kind of hard for me to handle. I was young and impressionable. I knew I wanted to do it so badly nobody could stop me, least of all people I wouldn't even bother to count as friends, but many times I did question it. I wondered why I was so different, why I wanted to do something a lot of people didn't like and even made fun of. If you played soccer, everybody loved you; you were a hero. And they gave you anything.

People recognized my athletic talents; but my choice of a sport confused them. They shook their heads. "Why did you have to pick the least-favorite sport in Austria?" they always asked. It was true. We had only twenty or thirty bodybuilders in the entire country.

I couldn't come up with an answer. I didn't know. It had been instinctive. I had just fallen in love with it. I loved the feeling of the gym, of working out, of having muscles all over.

Now, looking back, I can analyze it more clearly. My total involvement had a lot to do with the discipline, the individualism, and the utter integrity of bodybuilding. But at the time it was a mystery even to me. Bodybuilding did have its rewards, but they were relatively small. I wasn't competing yet, so my gratification had to come from other areas. In the summer at the lake I could surprise everyone by showing up with a different body. They'd say, "Jesus, Arnold, you grew again. When are you going to stop?"

"Never," I'd tell them. We'd all laugh. They thought it amusing. But I meant it.

It wasn't only my friends at school and the lake who were impressed. The neighbors, too, began giving me special attention. "If you need fresh milk, just tell us," a neighbor would say. "I know for lifting weights you need milk." Or eggs, or vegetables. Suddenly everyone around began regarding me as different. No matter whether they liked it or not—they couldn't overlook it.

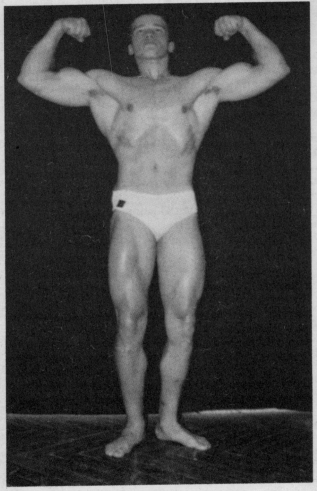

Studio poses at sixteen

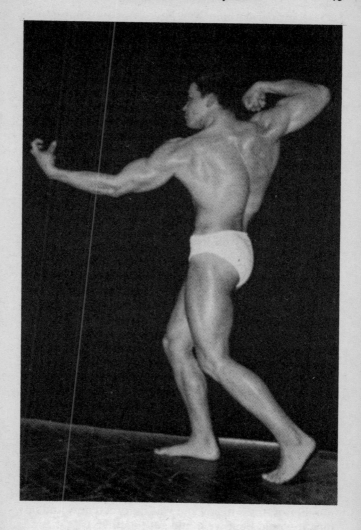

The strangest thing was how my new body struck girls. There were a certain number of girls who were knocked out by it and a certain number who found it repulsive. There was absolutely no in-between. It seemed cut and dried. I'd hear their comments in the hallway at lunchtime, on the street, or at the lake. "I don't like it. He's weird—all those muscles give me the creeps." Or, "I love the way Arnold looks—so big and powerful. It's like sculpture. That's how a man should look."

These reactions gave me added motivation to continue building my body. I wanted to get bigger so I could really impress the girls who liked it and upset the others even more. Not that girls were my main reason for training. Far from it. But they added incentive and I figured as long as I was getting this attention from them I might as well use it. I had fun. I could tell if a girl was repelled by my size. And when I'd catch her looking at me in disbelief, I would casually raise my arm, flex my bicep, and watch her cringe. It was always good for a laugh.

I remember there was one of these negative girls I wanted to date. Her name was Herta and I knew she claimed she wasn't turned on by my body. I wanted to try and change her mind. I pursued her and gradually we became friends. Finally one day I got up the nerve to ask her on a date. "I wouldn't go out with you in a million years," she said. "You're in love with yourself. You're in love with your own body. You look at yourself all the time. You pose in front of the mirror."

Her statement came like a slap in the face. At first I was angry. Why did she refuse to understand it? Why did she have to turn on me? But it was predictable. And I got over it. (I don't think she ever did, though. The last time I was in Graz for a visit, she called me a number of times to say she was divorced now and how nice it would be if we could get together.)

Nobody seemed to understand what was involved in bodybuilding. You do look at your body in a mirror, not because you are narcissistic, but because you are trying to check your progress. It has nothing to do with being in love with yourself. Herta would never have told one of the track stars he was in love with himself because he had someone check his speed with a stopwatch. It just happens that the mirror, the scales and the tape measure are the only tools a bodybuilder has for determining his progress.

Herta was hardly typical. I had no difficulty getting girls. I'd been introduced to sex with almost no hangups. The older bodybuilders at the gym had started including me in their parties. It was easy for me. These guys always saw to it that I had a girl. "Here, Arnold, this one's for you."

Girls became sex objects. I saw the other bodybuilders using them in this way and I thought it was all right. We talked about the pitfalls of romantic situations, serious ones, how it could take away from your training. Naturally, I agreed with them. They were my idols.

My attitude about all that has changed radically. I used to feel that women were here for one reason. Sex was simply another kind of exercise, another body function. I was convinced a girl and I couldn't communicate on equal footing because she wouldn't understand what I was doing. I didn't have time to take one girl out regularly and go through a normal high-school romance with all its phone calls and notes and squabbles. That took too much time. I needed to be in the gym. For me it was a simple matter of picking them up at the lake, and then never seeing them again. In fact it wasn't until four years after I started training that I had any meaningful communication with a girl.

I couldn't be bothered with girls as companions. My mind was totally locked into working out, and I was annoyed if anything took me away from it. Without making a conscious decision to do so, I closed a door on that aspect of growing up, that vulnerability, and became very protective of my emotions. I didn't allow myself to get involved—period. It wasn't a reasoned choice; it just happened out of necessity.

I started this practice early in my career and continued it for as long as it served to help me maintain a clear focus and drive myself toward a fixed point. This didn't mean I had no fun. I was only selfish and protective of that part of myself that people seemed always to want to get at in a relationship. And the more successful I became, the more strict I was in guarding it. I couldn't afford to have my feelings hurt during heavy training or just before a competition. I needed stable emotions, total discipline. I needed to be there training for two hours in the morning and two hours at night, concentrating on nothing except perfecting my body and bringing it to its peak.

Whatever I thought might hold me back, I avoided. I crossed girls off my list—except as tools for my sexual needs. I eliminated my parents too. It seemed they always wanted to see me, then when I was around they had nothing to say. I grew accustomed to hearing certain questions: "What's wrong with you, Arnold? Don't you feel anything? Don't you have any emotions?"

How can you answer that? I always let it pass with a shrug. I knew that what I was doing was not only justifiable, it was essential. Besides, if I did miss out on the emotional thing because I was so dedicated, I believe I benefited in other ways that finally brought everything into balance. One of these was my self-confidence, which grew as I saw how much control I was gaining over my body. In two or three years I had actually been able to change my body entirely. That told me something. If I had been able to change my body that much, I could also, through the same discipline and determination, change anything else I wanted. I could change my habits, my whole outlook on life.

During the early years I didn't care how I felt about anything except bodybuilding. It consumed every min-

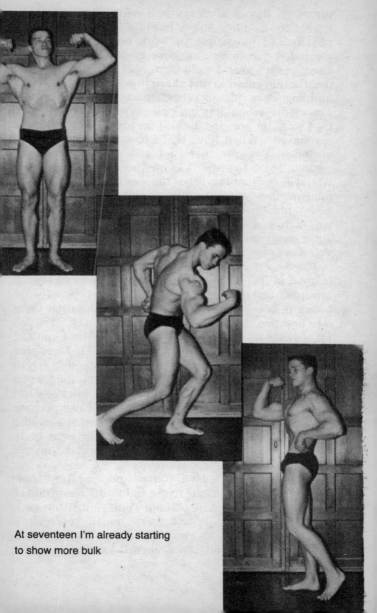

At seventeen I'm already starting
to show more bulk

ute of my days and all my best effort. But now that I train only an hour and a half a day to maintain my physique, I have time to work on the things I neglected. I can bring out those emotions I had to put away years ago and build them back into my life. I can use the information and discipline I learned in bodybuilding for perfecting other aspects of my life. Now if I catch myself holding back an emotion the way I used to, I work on bringing it out; I try to make myself more responsive. When I see that I have certain backward attitudes, I reason them out and work to make my outlook more realistic. I know there are some people who will say that this is not the way to do things. And I imagine they are the same people who always said bodybuilding was bad for your health. I proved that was wrong. I know that if you can change your diet and exercise program to give yourself a different body, you can apply the same principles to anything else.

The secret is contained in a three-part formula I learned in the gym: self-confidence, a positive mental attitude, and honest hard work. Many people are aware of these principles, but very few can put them into practice. Every day I hear someone say, "I'm too fat. I need to lose twenty-five pounds, but I can't. I never seem to improve." I'd hate myself if I had that kind of attitude, if I were that weak. I can lose ten to forty pounds rapidly, easily, painlessly, by simply setting my mind to it. By observing the principles of strict discipline that bodybuilding taught me, I can prepare myself for anything. I have developed such absolute control over my body that I can decide what body weight I want for any particular time and take myself up or down to meet it.

Two months before we started shooting *Stay Hungry,* Bob Rafaelson came to me and said, "I'm afraid of hiring you for this film, Arnold. You're just too goddamn big. You weigh two forty, and if you're in a scene with Sally Fields you'll dwarf her. I'd like you to be much leaner and more normal-looking in street clothes." I said, "You worry about your film and I'll worry about my body. Just tell me what day you want me to show up and at what body weight, and I'll do it." He thought I was pulling his leg. He wanted me to be down to 210 pounds, but he didn't think I could ever do it. So I bet him I could. The day the filming began, Rafaelson went with me to the gym to work out and take a sauna. "Step on the scale," he said. I weighed 209 pounds. One pound less than he wanted me. He couldn't believe it. I kept the weight for three months, until the shooting stopped. Then I got an offer to do the film *Pumping Iron*. The only way I could do it was to compete in the Mr. Olympia contest. Within two more months I would have to go back up to 240 pounds, the weight at which I felt I reached the ultimate in size and symmetry, and then cut down to 235 for maximum definition. I did it easily and won the Mr. Olympia contest.

From the very beginning I knew bodybuilding was the perfect choice for my career. No one else seemed to agree—at least not my family or teachers. To them the only acceptable way of life was being a banker, secretary, doctor, or salesman—being established in the ordinary way, taking the regular kind of job offered through an employment agency—something legitimate. My desire to build my body and be Mr. Universe was totally beyond their comprehension. Because of it, I was put through a lot of changes. I locked up my emotions even further and listened only to my inner voice, my instincts.

My mother, for one, didn't understand my drive at all. She had no time for sports. She couldn't even understand why my father kept training to stay in shape. But, strangely enough, she always had the attitude: "Let Arnold do what he wants. As long as he isn't a criminal, as long as he doesn't do anything bad, let him go on with his muscle building."

She changed her outlook as soon as I brought home my first weight-lifting trophy. She took it and ran from

house to house in Thal, the little village outside of
Graz where we lived, showing the neighbors what I
had won. It was a turning point for her. She began to
accept what I was doing. Now, all of a sudden, some
attention was focused on her. People singled her out:
this is the mother of the guy who just won the weight-
lifting championship, the mother of the strong man.
She too was treated as a champion. She was proud of
me. And then (up to a certain point) she encouraged
me to do what I wanted.

We still had our differences. She and my father were
Catholic. Every Sunday until I was fifteen, I went to
church with them. Then my friends started asking why
I did it. They said it was stupid. I had never given it
much thought one way or the other. It was a rule at
home: we went to church. Helmut Knaur, sort of an
intellectual among the bodybuilders, gave me a book
called *Pfaffenspiegel*, which was about priests, their
lives, how horrible they were, and how they'd altered
the history of the religion.

Reading that turned me completely around. Karl
and Helmut and I discussed it in the gym. Helmut
insisted that if I achieved something in life, I shouldn't
thank God for it, I should thank myself. It was the
same if something bad happened. I shouldn't ask God
for help, I should help myself. He asked me if I'd ever
prayed for my body. I confessed I had. He said if I
wanted a great body, I had to build it. Nobody else
could. Least of all God.

These were wild ideas for someone as young as I
was. But they made perfect sense and I announced to
my family that I would no longer go to church, that I
didn't believe in it and didn't have time to waste on it.
This added to the conflict at home.

Eventually there was a split between my parents
about me. My mother obviously knew what was going
on with me and the girls my friends lined up. She never
came out and said anything directly, but she let me
know she was concerned. Things were different be-

tween me and my father. He assumed that when I was eighteen, I would just go into the Army and they would straighten me out. He accepted some of the things my mother condemned. He felt it was perfectly all right to make out with all the girls I could. In fact, he was proud I was dating the fast girls. He bragged about them to his friends. "Jesus Christ, you should see some of the women my son's coming up with." He was showing off, of course. But still, our whole relationship had changed because I'd established myself by winning a few trophies and now had some girls. He was particularly excited about the girls. And he liked the idea that I didn't get involved. "That's right, Arnold," he'd say, as though he'd had endless experience, "never be fooled by them." That continued to be an avenue of communication between us for a couple of years. In fact, the few nights I took girls home when I was on leave from the Army, my father was always very pleasant and would bring out a bottle of wine and a couple of glasses.

My mother still wanted to protect me. We had to hide things from her. She was too religious; she imagined the awful state of my soul. And she felt sorry for the girls. To her it was all somehow connected with bodybuilding, and her antagonism for the sport grew. It bothered her that this had not merely been a phase of my growing up.

"You're lazy, Arnold!" she would shout. "Look at you. All you want to do is train with weights. That's all you think about. Look at your shoes," she would say, grasping at anything. "They're filthy. I've cleaned your father's because he's my husband. But I won't do yours. You can take care of yourself."

That aspect of it was getting to my father as well. The girls were all right. He liked that. And the trophies. He had a few of his own from ice curling, which we did together. But every so often he would take me aside and say, "Well, Arnold, what do you want to do?"

I would tell him again, "Dad, I'm going to be a professional bodybuilder. I'm going to make it my life."

"I can see you're serious," he would say, his eyes growing thoughtful. "But how do you plan to apply it? What do you want out of life?" A silence would grow between us. He would sigh, go back to his newspaper, and that would be the end of it until he felt compelled to question me again.

For a long time I would just shrug my shoulders and refuse to speak about it. Then one day when I was seventeen and had the plan more firmly in my own mind, I surprised him with a full reply. "I have two possibilities right now. One is that I can go into the Army, become an officer, and have some freedom to go on training." He nodded his head gravely. He felt I'd finally hit upon something. It would have made him proud for me to devote my life to the Austrian Army. "The other alternative is to go to Germany and then to America."

"America?" Now I was talking nonsense again.

I had already weighed out the good points of being an officer. The Austrian Army would give me schooling, food and clothing; then, as an athlete, I would be allowed unbelievable freedom. There was an elite military academy in Vienna that specialized in sports. They would equip a weight room for me; they would see that I had the best of everything.

My father and I talked more than once about that as my final goal. He looked at it as a career in the Army. I saw it as the means to an end—winning Mr. Universe. My father was concerned that I might be unable to earn a living from bodybuilding, that I would waste myself and my potential.

A career in the Army was my last choice. My real aspiration was to somehow get to America. I'd always had a claustrophobic feeling about Austria. "I've got to get out of here," I kept thinking. "It's not big enough, it's stifling." It wouldn't allow me to expand. There seemed never to be enough space. Even peo-

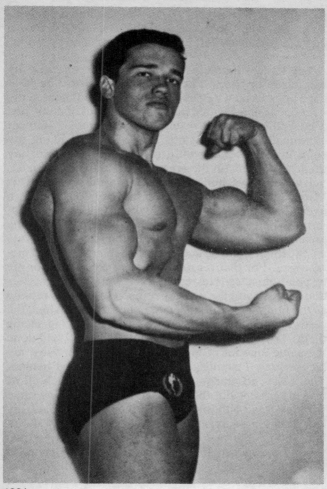

1964

ple's ideas were small. There was too much contentment, too much acceptance of things as they'd always been. It was beautiful; it was a great place to be old in.

Reg Park still dominated my life. I had changed my routine a few times. I kept the old exercises, the standard ones I knew Reg used. But I modified them to my own needs and I added new ones. Instead of doing just a barbell curl, I did a dumbbell curl too. I thought continually of making my biceps higher, giving my back thickness and width, increasing the size of my thighs. Working on the areas I wanted to emphasize.

I was always honest about my weak points. This helped me grow. I think it's the key to success in everything: be honest; know where you're weak; admit it. There is nobody in bodybuilding without some areas that need work. I had inherited from my parents an excellent bone structure and an almost perfect metabolism. For that reason it was basically easy for me to build muscles. However, there were some muscles that seemed stubborn. They refused to grow as rapidly as the others. I wrote them on note cards and stuck the cards around my mirror where I couldn't avoid seeing them. Triceps were the first I noted down. I had done the same amount of biceps and triceps exercises; my biceps grew instantly, but my triceps lagged behind. There was no reason for it. I had put as much effort into my triceps but they refused to respond. The same with my legs. Although I was doing a lot of squats, my legs didn't grow as rapidly as my chest. And my shoulders didn't improve as much as my back. After two years I could see that certain parts hadn't changed very much at all. I wrote them down and adjusted my workouts. I increased some exercises. I experimented. I watched my muscles for the results. Slowly I adjusted and evened out my body.

It was a long, almost unending process. At eighteen, I still didn't have my body equalized. There were weak points to work on. I was limited to what I knew and what was available locally to learn. I was held back severely by the Austrian mentality in bodybuilding, which was just to concentrate on big arms and a big chest, as though photographs would always be taken only from the waist up. Nobody I knew really considered the serrati or the intercostals, the muscles that give the body a look of finish, of quality. And that kind of provincial thinking was to hamper me for a long time to come.

I went into the Army in 1965. One year of service was obligatory in Austria. After that, I could make my decision about a future. For me the Army was a good experience. I liked the regimentation, the firm, rigid structure. The whole idea of uniforms and medals appealed to me. Discipline was not a new thing to me—you can't do bodybuilding successfully without it. Then too, I'd grown up in a disciplined atmosphere. My father always acted like a general, checking to see that I ate the proper way, that I did my studies.

His influence helped get me assigned as a driver in a tank unit. Actually I wasn't well-suited to be a tank driver; I was too tall and I was only eighteen (twenty-one was the minimum age), but it was something I badly wanted to do. The necessary strings were pulled and not only was I allowed to drive a tank, I was also stationed in a camp near Graz. That enabled me to continue training, which remained the most important part of my life.

Shortly after I was inducted, I received an invitation to the junior division of the Mr. Europe contest in Stuttgart, Germany. I was in the middle of basic training and our orders were to remain on the base for six weeks. Unless someone in your immediate family died, you were absolutely forbidden to leave. I spent a couple of sleepless nights wondering what I should do. Finally I knew there was no alternative: I was going to sneak out and go.

The junior Mr. Europe contest meant so much to me that I didn't care what consequences I'd have to suf-

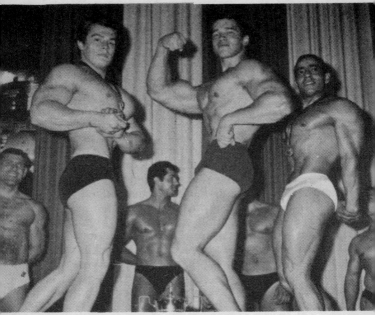

Winning my first competition, Mr. Europe Junior, 1965

fer. I crawled over the wall, taking only the clothes I was wearing. I had barely enough money to buy a third-class train ticket. It crept out of Austria into Germany, stopping at every station, and arrived a day later in Stuttgart.

This was my first contest. I was nervous and exhausted from the train trip and I had no idea what was going on. I tried to learn something by watching the short men's class, but they seemed as amateurish and confused as I was. I had to borrow someone else's posing trunks, someone else's body oil. I had rehearsed a posing routine in my mind on the train. It was a composite of all Reg Park's poses I'd memorized from the muscle magazines. But the instant I stepped out before the judges my mind went blank. Somehow I made it through the initial posing. Then they called me back for a pose-off. Again, my mind was blank and I wasn't sure how I'd done. Finally, the announcement came that I'd won—Arnold Schwarzenegger, Mr. Europe Junior.

When I look at the photographs that were taken then, I recall how I felt. The surprise wore off fast. I drew myself up. I felt like King Kong. I loved the sudden attention. I strutted and flexed. I knew for certain that I was on the way to becoming the world's greatest bodybuilder. I felt I was already one of the best in the world. Obviously, I wasn't even in the top 5,000; but in my mind I was the best. I had just won Mr. Europe Junior.

At first the Army was not impressed. I borrowed money to travel back to the base and they caught me as I was climbing over the wall. I sat in jail for seven days with only a blanket on a cold stone bench and almost no food. But I had my trophy and I didn't care if they locked me up for a whole year; it had been worth it.

I showed my trophy to everybody. And by the time I got out of jail, word had spread through the camp that I had won Mr. Europe Junior. The top majors decided it lent some prestige to the Army and gave me two days' leave. I became a hero because of what I'd gone through to win. When we were out in the field the drill instructors mentioned it. "You have to fight for your fatherland," they said. "You have to have courage. Look at what Schwarzenegger did just to win this title." I became a hero, even though I had defied their rules to get what I wanted. That one time, they made an exception.

In basic training, my bodybuilding gave me a tremendous boost; it put me way ahead of everyone else in physical prowess. And that, added to the notoriety I'd gained from winning Mr. Europe Junior, gave me a special status in the eyes of the officers. I went on to tank-driving school and loved driving those big machines and feeling the sturdy recoil of the guns when we fired. It appealed to the part of me that has always been moved by any show of strength and force. In the afternoons we cleaned and oiled the tanks. However, after a few days I was excused from those afternoon duties. An order came down from the top that I was to train, to build my body. It was the nicest order I could have had.

A weight-lifting gym was set up and I was ordered to go there every day after lunch. I'd brought my own dumbbells and some of the machines from home because the Army had only barbells and weights. They were strict about my training. Every time an officer walked by the window and caught me sitting down, he'd threaten to have me put in jail. That was his duty. If you got caught goofing off when you were supposed to be oiling and greasing the tanks, you'd be put away. The Army felt it was no different with what I was doing. I must train, they said, I must be lifting weights all the time.

I paced myself and used this opportunity to continue building the foundation I'd begun three years before. I devised a way of training six hours at a stretch without getting totally wiped out. I ate four or five times a day. They allowed me all the food I wanted; but in terms of nutrition, Army food wasn't worth much. It took a couple of pounds of the overcooked meat they served to provide the amount of protein you'd find in an average-sized medium-rare steak. Taking all this into consideration, I consumed huge quantities of food and then tried to burn off the extra calories.

Throughout the time I was in the Army I divided my training between bodybuilding and Olympic weight lifting. I was interested in lifting heavy weights over my head. The image of myself with a loaded barbell pressed up and my arms locked took a long time to get out of my system. Before I was eighteen, I had competed in the Austrian championships, winning first place in the heavyweight division. But after the Mr. Europe Junior contest I stopped Olympic lifting. It wasn't what I wanted to do. I'd done it primarily to prove a point—that a bodybuilder not only *looked* strong, he *was* strong, and that well-developed muscles were not merely ornamentation.

Many people regret having to serve in the Army. But it was not a waste of time for me. When I came out I weighed 225 pounds. I'd gone from 200 to 225 pounds. Up to that time, this was the biggest change I'd ever made in a single year.

Chapter Three

After I won the Mr. Europe Junior contest, one of the judges, a man I will call Schneck, who owned a gymnasium and a magazine in Munich, took me aside and said, "Schwarzenegger, you have a real talent for bodybuilding. You'll be the next great thing in Germany. As soon as you're out of the Army, I'd like you to come to Munich and manage my health and bodybuilding club. You can train as much as you want. Next fall I'll even pay your way to London to watch the Mr. Universe contest."

"What do you mean, *watch?*"

"You can watch the Mr. Universe contest," he repeated. "You can watch those guys and get inspired."

"Watch?" The word stuck in my mind.

He gave me a funny look. "You don't think—"

"Yes," I said. "I'm going over there and compete."

"No, no, no," he said and laughed. "You can't do that. Those guys are big bulls. They're big animals—so huge you wouldn't believe it. You don't want to compete against them. Not yet."

He talked as though they were years and years ahead of me. But as far as I was concerned, he had promised me a trip to London to the contest, and I was going to do what I wanted. "If I go over there, I'm going to compete," I told him, "not to watch."

He laughed and said, "Sure."

Munich was ideal for me. It was exciting, one of the fastest cities in middle Europe. Everything there seemed to be happening at once. It was big, with this feeling of wealth and power and barely contained energy; it seemed on the point of exploding. Even before I was settled and secure, I could see a future for myself. I could grow and expand. For the first time, I felt I could really breathe.

But the day I arrived from Austria, I was overwhelmed. Inside the train station I encountered a flood of foreign languages—Italian, French, Greek, German, Spanish, English, Dutch, Portuguese. There was no one to meet me: I had only an address to find. Each time I turned to someone to ask directions, I was met with a shrug and a statement that either they didn't speak German or they were strangers themselves. I carried my bags out of the station. Again, I couldn't believe it. I had never seen so many people. There were crowds and crowds of people and they all seemed to be hurrying somewhere. Endless lines of cars honked and sped past. Buildings rose up close and tall.

I remember turning around slowly, looking at it all and saying to myself, "There's no way back now, Arnold."

Of course, I knew I would never want to go back. I was meant to be there, and to go on. The plan I'd begun formulating three years ago was beginning to work.

I went to Munich fresh, naive, and pretty innocent. I was a big Austrian kid from a small country village and I was impressed with everything about this teeming city. I couldn't get enough of it. Schneck, my new employer, drove me around in his Mercedes. He showed me all the things he owned, including his beautiful house, where he had promised I could have a room.

I stayed with him for three or four days. I did have a separate room, but there was no bed in it. I slept on a couch, which was uncomfortable for someone my size. Schneck promised he would get a bed: he said

one had been ordered. It never arrived, of course, and
he finally suggested that I should sleep in his bedroom.

I got the message. It went up my spine like a sudden
chill. I packed my clothes and left the house.

He followed me outside. "Think about it, Arnold,"
he said, stopping me. "You wouldn't be the first one."
He told me about two other bodybuilders who had
stayed with him. "Look where they are now. They've
got their own gymnasiums. They've got an easy life,
Arnold."

"No," I said. As tough and firm as I meant to sound,
I remember being a little bit frightened. I was trem-
bling inside. Partly it was from fear, but mostly it was
rage.

Schneck had always seemed so smooth and sure of
himself. Now I saw that he was sweating. He leaned
close. "You know I can get you into films. I can
finance you while you train for Mr. Universe. Later I'll
send you to America, to California, to train with the
big champions." He painted this clever picture based
on all the things I'd told him I wanted to do with my
life. I did want a health club and a career in the
movies, the kind of life Reg Park had had. I wanted to
go to America and train with the top musclemen.
America was in my head always. It was the mecca of
bodybuilding. The champions always seemed to go to
America. And that impressed me more than any of his
arguments.

I thought about it. I actually considered it, which
was not so astonishing. Schneck was a pro. He knew
how to manipulate young guys with their heads full of
dreams.

"Just come back inside, Arnold," he coaxed. "Let's
not talk on the street."

I went inside with him. I sat in a chair and listened to
more of his talk. He reiterated everything he'd said,
making his promises all seem more attractive. I
watched him while he talked. I hated what I saw in his
eyes. Everything in me was saying no. I realized I
would get everything he promised eventually if I just

kept pushing myself. I wanted to do it with dignity. I wanted to do it in a good way, rather than have something I'd feel sorry about.

"No—" I said. I shook my head and got up.

He reached out to touch me.

"No—" I said.

He knew I meant it.

I continued to work in the gymnasium, but my relationship with Schneck wasn't good. We did finally become friends much later, when I no longer needed him for anything. But at first it was a strain. I had to see him almost daily and occasionally he would let me know that his offer still stood. I kept getting more and more independent. That made it easier for me to say no. And after a while I loosened up enough so I could even laugh about our encounter with my friends in the gym. I became aware of the fact that there were a few homosexuals around bodybuilding. These were not the bodybuilders themselves, not the serious ones. Two or three rich guys in Munich hung out in gyms and tried to pick up young bodybuilders by promising them the world. Some of them did accept. But I was never sorry I turned down the offers I had.

I found myself a room. I couldn't afford much. It was one of those places people let out when they have extra space in their apartment and want help paying the rent. You eat with them and share a bathroom.

My ego wouldn't allow me to let my parents know what a struggle I was having. As far as they knew, I was happy, earning a decent salary, and making progress in every direction. Otherwise they would have gotten on my case to come home.

At that point my own thinking was tuned in to only one thing: becoming Mr. Universe. In my own mind, I *was* Mr. Universe; I had this absolutely clear vision of myself up on the dais with the trophy. It was only a matter of time before the whole world would be able to see it too. And it made no difference to me how much I had to struggle to get there.

Managing a health club was an entirely new experi-

ence. I was supposed to be a trainer, to show people
how to exercise, to devise programs which would
make them lose fat and rebuild their bodies. At first,
confronted with these people who'd come to me for
guidance, I felt helpless. I thought I still needed
someone giving me advice on my workouts. But I
realized I had to do it in order to survive.

I had to live a split life, acting as an instructor to the
health club clients on the one hand, and trying to train
myself for the Mr. Universe title on the other. It was
frustrating. People who would never benefit from what
I told them kept taking my time. They paid and came
to the gym. But it was a disgusting, superficial effort
on their part. They merely went through the motions,
doing sissy workouts, pampering themselves. And
there was so much I wanted to do with those wasted
hours.

I trained both morning and evening. It was the beginning of the split routine that would later become
famous. But I got into it originally because it was expe-
dient. There was no initial theory involved. I worked
out from nine to eleven in the morning and then again
from seven to nine at night. I couldn't believe the results. Within two months I gained another five pounds.

In the Army, when I had trained six hours continuously, I found that I could never handle the kind of
weight I wanted to use. But by splitting up my
schedule, training arms and shoulders in the morning,
resting for a few hours and eating at least two substan-
tial six-course meals, then going back to train my legs,
chest and abdominals in the evening, I discovered I
had plenty of energy to handle a lot of poundage. It
was like a whole new workout on a different day. I was
rested, my energy was back, and my mind was ready
for it.

At first, nobody paid much attention to this split
routine, except to knock it. They thought I was stupid
to train twice a day. They said I'd get overtrained, that
my muscles would start to deteriorate.

I ignored them. I kept pushing myself and growing, growing fast. I had two immediate goals. I was going to win Mr. Europe and I was going to compete in a Mr. Universe contest. I felt good about the Mr. Europe; it was a cinch. But I had no idea how I'd do in London. At that point I no longer knew how I'd get to London. Schneck had taken back his offer and I didn't have the money myself. But I knew I'd make it somehow. And I didn't know how big those guys would be. People kept telling me they were gigantic, they were animals, monsters. All I had to judge by were photographs—which I knew could be deceptive. I looked at the guys who had competed in the previous contest. "No," I decided, "I can't beat the guy who won." I'd look at the second-place winner. "No, I can't beat him." I'd look at the guy who placed third. "I can't beat him either." I went right down the line, trying to figure out who I might beat. I got to eighth or ninth place and figured I might have a chance if I tried hard enough.

It was a loser's way of looking at it. I defeated myself before I even entered, before I'd even completed the year's training. But I was young. I was being self-protective. I hadn't yet pulled together my ideas about positive thinking and the powers of the mind over the muscles.

At the Mr. Europe contest, rumors about me were circulating long before I arrived. People were anxious to get a look at this monster from Munich. They had heard all these stories from the bodybuilding circuit. "Arnold has nearly fifty centimeters of arm . . . " (Which was close to 20 inches.) The most amazing thing about that was my age: "Arnold is only nineteen years old . . . " Nobody could figure it out at all. People at the contest crowded around me. They wanted to look, to touch. "How did you do it?" they asked. They were flipped out. They thought I must be training under some special drug program or something.

Onstage, the first pose I did was double biceps— because I knew my greatest strength was arms. The judges almost fainted. When I hit the first arm shot, they looked at me with their mouths hanging open. I flexed again and heard one judge whisper, "Oh, my god, where'd this guy come from?" After hearing his comment, there was no stopping me. I felt as if my body were blooming, unfolding, opening up. I filled up with energy and kept posing, doing ten times more poses than I had intended. I just didn't want to leave the platform.

I experienced something I had never felt before: a rush of confidence, a feeling I was going to win. It seemed to sweep me up and carry me along with it. I noticed, too, that the judges picked up on it. I did win. I wiped out all the favorites. In fact, I made such an impression on the officials that they decided to pay my ticket to the Mr. Universe contest.

A week later, I entered the competition for the Best Built Man of Europe. I won that one too. But it backfired on me. It was not sponsored by the same federation as the Mr. Europe contest and that first federation declared I had violated something in their code and was therefore no longer eligible for the ticket to the Mr. Universe contest.

What a blow that was. The owner of the gymnasium had backed out, and the Mr. Europe people had disqualified me because I'd entered and won another contest. I couldn't believe it.

I was dejected, naturally, but I had too much drive to let this political maneuvering stop me. I wasn't alone in my efforts. Reinhart Smolana, who owned another gymnasium in Munich, recognized how hungry I was for winning and got behind me. Reinhart knew what it was all about. The year before, he had competed and won his height class at the Mr. Universe contest. However, he realized he would never win the overall award because he didn't have enough body weight. So he started a collection and put all his energy into trying to get me to London. And finally, after one

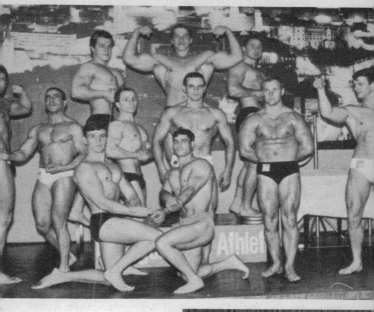

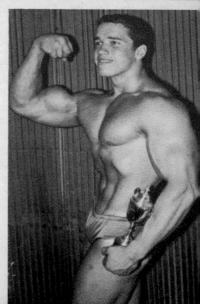

Winning Mr. Europe, 1966

solid month of hassling and scraping, we had enough money for a ticket.

That was the first time I'd ever flown anyplace. I was on my way to the Mr. Universe contest and I had never even been in an airplane. Which is just one more indication of how inexperienced I was. I hadn't been willing to work my way up through the countless little Mr. Thises and Mr. Thats. I was shooting for the top.

I remember thinking as I did up my seat belt, "What if it crashes and I never get there?" And when I heard the landing gear come up with a shudder into the body of the plane, it was like a cold fist closing on my heart. I was certain we were gone.

I arrived in London knowing almost no English. I kept repeating, "I would like to go to the Royal Hotel, please," a sentence I had practiced during the flight. Two businessmen from Munich said they were staying at the Royal and took me in their taxi.

When we got there, I didn't see any bodybuilders. Something was wrong. Where was the Mr. Universe contest? The businessmen asked at the desk and then translated for me. The contest was at another Royal Hotel.

I ran back to the taxi with the correct address. There was no mistake this time. As we pulled up at the curb, I saw at least fifty huge guys standing outside the glass doors. They seemed to be waiting for something. They were monstrous, wearing jackets padded out to almost twice the width of their actual shoulders. There were dudes with funny haircuts from India and Africa, guys wearing clothes from all different parts of the world.

As soon as I stepped out of my cab they started moving toward me. They crowded close, grabbing and feeling my arms and talking in at least ten different languages. Apparently they had all been waiting for me. They had heard I was the first bodybuilder in Europe with 20-inch arms. In America that measurement wasn't unusual, but in Europe it was phenomenal—especially on someone barely nineteen years old.

People hung around me all day. Their minds were blown by my size, by the size of my arms. I was like a little kid with all this attention. I didn't know what to do, how to act. I wanted to stay in the background and learn. That was the main reason I had come. But nobody would allow it.

My own eyes were popping. It was the first time I had seen blacks with frizzy hair. And I wondered how anybody could have shoulders as wide as the guys whose jackets stood out like building girders. (Later I learned the answer. When they took them off there was nothing underneath. One Frenchman even had a metal frame built into his.)

All that year, training for the Mr. Universe contest, I had not seriously expected to win (which was a kind of thinking I was never again to accept from myself): I'd somehow convinced myself I merely wanted to go and see what a big *international* competition was all about. Of course, somewhere in the back of my mind, hardly more solidly formulated than a daydream, was the idea that *maybe* I could win. But it was nothing more than that.

Then all of a sudden in London I found myself being admired by almost every bodybuilder there. This did something positive to me. I started thinking it really might be possible for me to win. That feeling I'd had at the Mr. Europe contest, that flood of self-confidence, started to come again. I felt stronger, I felt ready. I began walking differently, giving out bits of advice in my limited English, allowing my body to open up and my muscles to show even under my clothes.

I knew that the guys who were admiring my arms, making such a fuss over me, were no threat. So I broke away from them and went around the hotel to size up the rest of my competition. The pictures I'd seen in the magazines during the year hadn't told me half the truth about a few of them. But with all the attention I'd been getting, I began to feel I could beat them all.

That idea vanished the first time I saw Chet Yorton. He was coming out of an elevator I was waiting to get in. I stepped back, almost with amazement, and got this sudden sinking feeling: something inside me said there was no way I could beat this man. I admitted it and accepted defeat in that instant. Yorton had come over as the top favorite from America. The magazines already said he had the title as good as won, it was merely a matter of going through the motions. He was absolutely fantastic. He had a different look, a smooth, supple look I had not expected.

I had thought that 230 pounds of body weight and a 20-inch arm would easily get me to the top. But one look at Chet Yorton told me big arms and a massive body would never be enough. A winner had to have a specific look, a winning look. And Yorton had that look. He was golden brown; he was cut up, defined, each muscle thoroughly mapped with veins. This was the first time I realized the value of being able to see veins on the body. Veins are not particularly attractive to look at, but they tell you a great deal about your condition, about how much or how little fat you have. If you have a layer of fat between your skin and your muscles, you will show no veins. Seeing Yorton told me one thing: Arnold, you are fat. I knew I had to get veins. Which was a new thing for me.

Compared to most of us in Europe, Chet Yorton and the other Americans were like special creations of science. Their bodies seemed totally ready—finished, polished. Mine was far from finished. I had just come to London with a big, muscular body. And I suddenly saw myself at the beginning of another long, long road, one I'd have to travel if I ever expected to win. The kind of thing I was seeing there had very little to do with body size, which was what I had concentrated on. That was mere foundation material. Now I had to work it down, to carve and shape it. I had to get the separation, the finish, the tan.

Backstage before the contest I heard endless theories. Some guys were talking about taking saunas before competition as a way of wringing the last bit of water out of their systems. Some were claiming that tensing and flexing helped promote great definition and vascularity. I kept hearing new things right and left. I understood only enough English to get it in snatches, which made it even more confusing. Then another bodybuilder finally started translating for me, and I realized this was not a sport but a very complex science. I had assumed that after almost five years of training I knew all there was to know about bodybuilding; as it turned out, I knew next to nothing.

Usually, a bodybuilding contest is held on two different days, one afternoon and the following evening. The prejudging—which is the *real* judging—takes place on the first afternoon; the show the public attends is in the evening and is more a simple awarding of the titles. The first event is a relatively solemn affair attended only by a select audience. This is normally made up of the press, other bodybuilders and federation officials. The judges call out the lineup from each of the three classes—short, medium and tall men, in that order. They consider them in a group and individually. Their scores are made on judging sheets, which are kept secret until the next evening, when the class winners are announced and the overall winner is named from the top three. Although nothing can be certain at the prejudging, it is possible to get a fairly accurate reading on how things are going from the reactions of this knowledgeable audience. And that day at the Royal Hotel I felt I was definitely doing well—better than I had ever hoped. Everyone came up afterward to talk to me. They seemed to be trying to tell me I had something special.

When I took my place in the lineup of the tall men, I noticed something strange. Although I was the tallest, I held the next-to-last number. Chet Yorton had registered late—so his name was last on the list. I remember thinking it was a trick, a typical American trick, because the last one in line is the last one to pose; and that person has the advantage of making the last impression. Yes, it was just another American trick. I was sure of it.

Having seen Yorton, I didn't expect much from the competition. However, as soon as I went on I got a burst of applause. People were genuinely impressed. I was Mr. Europe, I had such big arms, and I was young, incredibly young.

I was really inexperienced about the finer points of competition. I had no idea what pose to hit for what effect. Most of my posing routine, if it could be called that, was still copied from what I had seen other bodybuilders doing or poses I had seen in magazines. It was not planned as it ought to have been, with the kind of unity and rhythm that would make the poses show off my body to its best advantage.

The actual show for the general public was held the next evening at the Victoria Palace Theatre. Again, there was a lot of confusion backstage. I was trying to get pumped up, trying to concentrate on my body, and also trying to absorb as much as I could of what was going on, what was being said.

The announcer gave me an enthusiastic introduction: "And now, ladies and gentlemen, allow me to introduce the new sensation from Germany, Mr. Europe, Arnold Schwarzenegger. He is nineteen, already a fantastic top bodybuilder, and this is his first time in an international competition. Let's give him a great welcome." The applause was so loud and persistent it was impossible to hear the last of his statement.

I had never appeared before so many people. The theater held nearly 3,000 and it was filled. I was afraid I would freeze up, that I wouldn't be able to pose at all. To avoid that, I fixed my gaze on a light high up in the ceiling. I hit my first pose and people screamed. There it was again, that warm rush through my body. I started opening up. I struck another pose and people applauded more. I kept posing and they kept applauding. I knew my time was running out, but I didn't want to get off the platform. I just focused on this white light somewhere up in the top of the theater and went through my clumsy posing routine. When I left the stage, the applause wouldn't stop.

"Go on, Arnold," someone said. And they pushed me back onstage. Up to that point, I was the only one who'd had to do an encore. In my nineteen years of life, I had not experienced anything that meant as much to me as those three minutes of posing. I told myself that it made the entire four years of training worthwhile.

Then Chet Yorton went out. I was fascinated watching him pose. He was totally in control, confident, strong. His whole appearance was rugged and virile. For the first time I was witnessing the real winning attitude in action. I could see that he felt like a winner. He was formidable. He had been known around Europe as the man to watch, the man who would come in one day and beat everybody. He'd won Mr. California, he'd won Mr. America twice, and had trophies for all the body parts—best legs, best calves, best back— everything. He had just finished making a film with Dave Draper called *Don't Make Waves,* which made him a movie star; and now he'd been sent to London to win this contest. All these things together prepared him mentally for a victory. You could see that in the easy way he moved across the stage: confidence seemed to ooze from his pores.

Yorton didn't have what I would call a flowing posing routine. He ripped his poses off like a machine. Each one was just: *bang!* A number of the men in the smaller classes had smooth routines which made them look beautiful and fluid as they moved from one pose to another. But between Yorton's poses there was nothing. There was just each pose. And you knew exactly what you were supposed to look at in each pose. He hammered them off one after another. He kept every muscle tensed, every muscle under control. His facial expressions were proud and relaxed. They always expressed one attitude: *I am the winner.*

It was also the first time I realized how important it was to flex your legs when you posed. I wasn't tuned in to legs. I was still hung up with the Austrian idea that chest and arms were everything—in spite of having chosen Reg Park as my idol.

Yorton seemed to know all the little tricks. He had certain leg and foot positions that caused his calves to pop out like diamonds. In one double biceps pose he did a little twist with his hips that made his waist appear inches smaller. Another biceps pose he did not do in the regular way, with the fists in; he turned the fists out to show his forearm as well as his bicep.

I ended up in second place. I knew I never could have beaten Yorton. He had all the qualities it took to be Mr. Universe—the muscularity, the separation, the definition, the skin color, the glow of confidence. He was finished, like a piece of sculpture ready to be put on display, complete with the patina.

As always, once I was over the initial disappointment of losing, I began trying to understand exactly why I had lost. I tried to be honest, to analyze it fairly. Aside from my total lack of finish, I still had some serious weaknesses. I had come to the contest with something good, but not good enough to win. I had a lot of mass, a great rough cut. My weak points were calves and thighs. I needed to work on posing, on diet, and all the finer points of bodybuilding.

For me, that was a real turning point. I decided I had to go back and spend a year on things I had never really given any time to at all. Once I'd mastered them, I knew I'd be on my way to being a winner.

A number of people recognized this in me. After the contest they came around and talked about Steve Reeves, how he had won the title at twenty-three, how he'd been the youngest person ever. They said I would beat that record. "Next year you'll win, Arnold. You'll be the youngest Mr. Universe in history." I knew they were right. Next year I would be Mr. Universe.

But I didn't look at it as a sure thing. I would have to go through a lot of changes in the next year. I knew the standards of bodybuilding were steadily moving up. Bodybuilders were becoming better and better. I'd seen the sport improve by leaps and bounds in the few years since I'd begun training. In 1962 Joe Abender, the Mr. Universe winner of that year, had 18½-inch arms. The same with Tommy Samsone in 1963. But now the 19-inch arm wasn't even big enough to get you in the top five. I'd come in second with 20-inch arms. Next year it would take even more. I had no idea what surprises would be coming from America. It was a crazy country with a seemingly endless supply of potential champions. Every year there was someone new from America, someone fantastic.

I was relying on one thing. What I had more than anyone else was drive. I was hungrier than anybody. I wanted it so badly it hurt. I knew there could be no one else in the world who wanted this title as much as I did.

Writers from the American muscle magazines came to me in the dressing room and asked for an interview. I thought they were joking. I laughed. "No, Arnold," my interpreter said. "They're serious."

They turned on tape recorders and had their photographers shoot pictures. They wanted to know how I trained, what were my secrets. I didn't feel I had any secrets. I needed to *know* the secrets. What was going on? They kept questioning me. I talked about the basic exercises, my split routine for training.

Finally I asked them how the champions in America trained. Then they thought I was joking. But I wanted to know. I could have asked Chet Yorton a thousand questions. I knew he lived in California, the mecca of bodybuilding. He trained with the top bodybuilders, Dave Draper, Larry Scott, the guys at the very top. He was only twenty-eight but he was considered an expert. From the way he looked and acted, I thought he must know everything. I asked him only a few questions. I didn't want him thinking I was just picking his brain so I could win the title next year. Primarily, I was interested in legs. What did he do that was different? The exercises he named were not in themselves different, but the way he did them was. His number of repetitions was higher. This helped separate the muscles and burn in the cuts.

I had thought perhaps he had some special exercises, but that wasn't true. He concentrated on the standard exercises. That was his "secret"—concentration. He worked to get everything an exercise could give him.

Being around Yorton backstage for a few minutes made me painfully aware of my own shortcomings. Aside from my weak legs, I hadn't trained my abdominals and I showed none of the quality muscles, such as serrati, which make a nice little studding between the pectoral and the latissimus. My weakest important point was legs. I had built big thighs, but I couldn't flex them. I couldn't show any definition: my legs were like two huge clumps. I had trained my calves, but not correctly—and certainly not with a fraction of the effort I put into the rest of my body. Yorton was training his thighs and calves as seriously as his arms and chest. Although I was constantly flexing my chest and arms, I rarely bothered about flexing my leg biceps, and I never thought about trying to control my calf muscles.

When I'd left for London, my friends and I, all the people who had contributed toward my ticket, thought it would be fantastic if I placed even in the top six. We discussed it in those terms and decided that doing so well in the first contest would be a clear indication that someday I could actually win the title. When they heard I'd come in second, they were ecstatic. Their minds were blown. They picked me up at the airport and rushed me into Munich for a big victory celebration. We had everything imaginable to drink—in kegs, bottles, cans. There was wild music and dancing. But there was just one thing in my mind: I couldn't wait to get to the gym and start working for next year's contest.

Chapter Four

I returned immediately to my training schedule. I didn't lay off at all. Twice a day, religiously, I put everything else out of my mind and did my workouts.

Other things began happening for me, things that would eventually affect the shape of my whole life. The man who owned the health club I had been managing suddenly announced he was ready to get out of the gymnasium business. He wanted to continue only publishing his magazine and manufacturing protein. He offered the business to me first. It was the perfect opportunity. I would be able to train and be independent. I couldn't ask for anything better. But I didn't have the money to buy the equipment. I could borrow some of it, but not enough. I was not established enough to go to a bank, and my friends had almost no money. I knew somehow I had to find the money. And I did—managing other clubs, selling food supplements, giving private lessons, and doing whatever odd jobs I could pick up.

With these and the sums I was able to borrow from friends, I was finally able to scrape together enough to buy the gym equipment. Even then things did not let up. I still had the loans to repay and there were improvements that had to be made in the gym. It was a struggle, a hell of a struggle.

I didn't let my family know about these troubles. They had no idea what was going on. They were upset

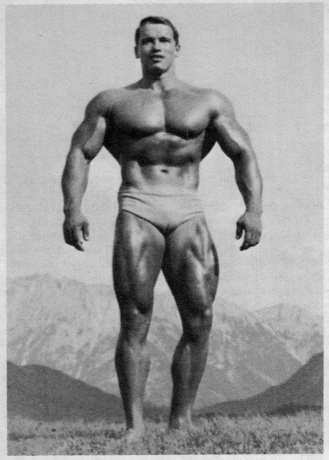

At nineteen, in the Bavarian Alps, one week before placing second in the Mr. Universe contest about my going from the Army to Munich, leaving home to manage a gymnasium and refusing to go on to school and prepare myself for some respectable profession. They called me periodically and wrote letters. They asked when I was going to get a real job, when I was going to become stable. "Is this what we raised," they asked, "a bum?" "How long will you go on training all day in a gymnasium and living in a dream world?" I endured all this negative thinking. Every time I visited home for a holiday, my mother would take me aside and say, "Why don't you listen to your father, Arnold? Use him as an example. Look what he's done with his life. He has accomplished things. He's with the police. He's respected."

I let everything they said pass over my head. My thinking went totally beyond that, beyond jobs, beyond Austria and small-town respectability. I continued doing precisely what I knew I needed to do. In my mind, there was only one possibility for me and that was to go to the top, to be the best. Everything else was just a means to that end.

My parents had no idea how closely I was having to live during my early period in Munich or they'd have been even more insistent.

One thing that saved me was my interest in business. I had majored in it in high school. I think somewhere in the back of my mind I realized I would have to have a good understanding of the mechanics of business in order to make my dreams profitable. I began putting this to use in Munich. I turned the publicity from having placed second in the Mr. Universe contest to attracting new members to my gym. In almost no time I built the membership from 70 to 200.

Then, shortly after I returned to Germany, I competed in a contest in Essen. Because of my performance at the Mr. Universe contest, I was treated as a Superman. I don't think the judges even bothered to look critically at me. I had the contest won the moment I walked through the door. Although it's not customary to do any measuring during a competition, one of the judges took out a tape and measured my arm, which was over 20 inches. That was it for him, that was all he was concerned about.

I went back to Munich with still more coverage in the bodybuilding press. That brought an even bigger increase of membership in my gym. Things were finally beginning to look better. I could pay my debts and still have money left for myself.

Later that fall I received a letter from London asking if I would come to England to do an "exhibition." Within days another one came from Newcastle, one from Plymouth, one from Portsmouth and another from Belfast—all asking me to do "exhibitions." I was bewildered. What did they mean by "exhibitions"? I didn't understand that side of bodybuilding at all.

The London letter was from Wag Bennett, who had been one of the Mr. Universe judges. He had invited me to his house for dinner after the contest was over and told me he liked my type of body more than Yorton's; he had, in fact, put me in first place. He had arranged the London show and had been instrumental in encouraging the other promoters on the English circuit to invite me. He informed me that he and his family would like to help, to advise me on my posing routine. I remembered that I'd felt comfortable with Bennett and wrote back to accept his offer.

I flew to London a few days prior to the exhibition. Wag put me up in his house and proceeded to teach me to pose to music. At first I was indignant. I had won second place in the Mr. Universe contest. I thought, What makes him think he can show me how to pose?

It was a stupid, arrogant reaction. The truth is, I could not have had a better or more understanding teacher. Wag Bennett had been judging contests for many years and knew a great deal about what was impressive both to judges and to an audience. In the living room, he gave me some initial instruction about what constituted effective posing. I didn't want to take off my shirt. I wanted to wait and surprise him with how much I had improved since the contest the month before. When I did strip down to my trunks, he was impressed. And he said it was all the more reason to put together a dynamic posing routine, using music.

I was totally confused by his suggestion that I pose to music. I didn't have an ear for music, and I didn't like the semi-classical stuff he said I ought to use. At the time, I thought anything old or classical was boring, a waste of time. I liked up-to-date music, something popular, with a beat, something that moved. He explained that for the purpose of the exhibition I had to use more complex music which had depth and texture. The record he felt would give me the range I needed was the sound track from the movie *Exodus*.

Wag explained something I understood but had never bothered to formulate myself. Bodybuilding was show business, especially in its advanced stages of competition and exhibition. If I expected to make it big in the field, I had to become a showman. Naturally, that argument sold me.

He put on the music from *Exodus*. At first, I was embarrassed. I had to laugh. I couldn't pose to that. He urged me to try. He showed me how to hit the best, most dramatic poses during the high points of the music and how to do the less dramatic, more subtle poses during the quieter parts. He taught me to move and turn with rhythm and flow. He brought out photographs of other bodybuilders in action and ran films of them posing. He explained why some of them worked and others didn't. After two days, I ended up with an entirely different posing routine.

In the beginning, I'm not sure Wag thought I would be able to do it. As big as I was, and as uncertain, I imagine I looked clumsy and slow. Plus I probably showed very little progress. I'm never that good when I practice anything. It's only when I'm really doing it, when it has to count, that I turn on. Which happened in London at the first exhibition. The moment I

stepped out on stage, everything fell into place. The
results amazed me. It all happened as Wag had predicted. The people applauded when the music was up,
and when it was down they were quiet. The whole
thing worked. After I'd finished, the audience kept
cheering and applauding and I realized the music had
done it. Before, my posing had been like a silent film
and now it was a sound film. It gave me a whole new
dimension. The lights were special to create shadows
on the body, the music starting and stopping dramatically; I felt as though I were having something
created for me, something very satisfying. I was up on
a pedestal with 2,000 people watching and I felt great.

That night I signed autographs for the first time. I
couldn't believe it. People crowded around me and
shoved papers in my hand. I didn't know what to do
with them. "Sign them!" cried Wag. "They want your
autograph." What a feeling that was to write *Arnold
Schwarzenegger* across the program. All of a sudden I
was a star.

Now bodybuilding did become show business for
me. I boughtExodus and took it everywhere I went. I
acted like a real professional, bringing my own music,
telling the stage manager what lights to use and when
to open and close the curtains. That's my style. As
soon as I grasp something, I take control.

The response to these exhibitions throughout Great
Britain was fabulous. The Dutch heard about them and
asked me to come to Holland. They didn't want just
any bodybuilder. Even though I was a newcomer, they
wanted Arnold. It had to do with having a big body,
being spectacular. People could identify more closely
with a huge body than with a perfect body. In those
days, a perfect body was too advanced. People could
relate to hugeness, to the animal spectacle of a big guy.
They called me "The Giant of Austria" and "The Austrian Oak." Articles read: "if Hercules were to be born
today his name would be Arnold Schwarzenegger."

I did an exhibition in Holland, one in Belgium, then
went back to England. I was paid 100 marks plus ex-

penses for each exhibition. It was almost nothing but I was happy. I still had no money to speak of. But I was young. I knew there was money in my future. I was getting experience doing these exhibitions. I learned all the little gimmicks—that I should smile, not look too serious, oil myself carefully, and limit the number of poses to keep the fans shouting for more.

I was becoming a pro. Already my actions were beyond my years and experience. I was growing so fast, moving ahead and becoming so suddenly famous in bodybuilding that I could barely watch what was happening to me.

I trained hard that whole year. I kept training the same way, using the split routine—which I was no longer doing out of necessity. Now a lot of other bodybuilders started following this routine. American magazines wrote about the split routine as if it were my secret; it became the big thing. Everybody thought that was how I'd grown as much as I had in such a short time.

Although the gym was a burden, I could see that it would be profitable. I struggled through, paying my debts, making ends meet.

I started having a good time in Munich. I met some bodybuilders who were serious about training. I was becoming a star, being interviewed and photographed, and I let that go to my head. I was young, full of energy, and began running wild. I got into powerlifting and trained with Franco Columbu. I turned Franco on to bodybuilding and he turned me on to powerlifting, on to heavy resistance training, which is different from bodybuilding. I liked the idea of really pressing a lot of weight, so I started competing in powerlifting events. Besides the ego satisfaction I got from working with heavy weights, it gave my body more mass, which I still felt I needed. It was an idea I couldn't get out of my head. I was doing heavy squats, heavy bench presses, and this provided some of the foundation work of my body, which has always made me appear strong. Certain bodybuilders lack that look. They have good bodies but they don't appear powerful. The reason is inadequate foundation training. Good early training shows up in the muscles around the spine. There is really no exercise for those muscles; their development is just an indication that you have put in some heavy ground work, heavy squats and heavy dead lifts, a lot of lifting and rowing. I had done these exercises from the start. I developed strong basic muscles which gave me the powerful look people wanted to see.

Reg Park had been a powerlifter; he had done squats with 600 pounds, bench presses with 500 pounds, and dead lifts of over 700 pounds. I saw no reason why I shouldn't continue in the same groove. I won the German championships in heavy-weight powerlifting before I stopped. My body weight was up to 250 and I convinced myself that it was time to chisel down, to start getting more quality in my body.

I met Reg Park in January of 1967. After winning second in the Mr. Universe contest, I began writing letters to him. Before that, when I was just a young bodybuilder, a nobody, I hadn't been sure he would bother to answer. But now he did write back, saying he had indeed heard of me and was looking forward to meeting me sometime. He said he was doing a show in London at the beginning of the year and suggested that we might meet then. I wrote to Wag Bennett and asked if there was any way I could do the exhibition with Reg Park.

I remember training in the gym in London and hearing he would be arriving there in an hour. I kept training and getting more and more excited. I was like a child. I was going to meet my idol for the first time. I felt giddy. I increased the weight on the barbell. I looked at myself in the mirror. I kept working—as if I could finish my body before he arrived. I wanted to be pumped up; I wanted to be at my best. I was very nervous about it. My mind was churning.

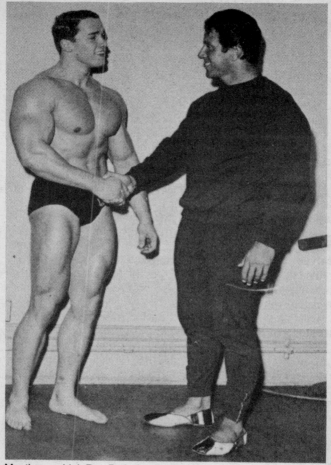

Meeting my idol, Reg Park, for the first time

Then he walked in the door. It was really incredible
seeing my idol for the first time. I recall having this
foolish self-conscious smile on my face. I just kept
looking at him and smiling—almost like when a girl has
a crush on a boy and she doesn't know what to say;
she just has this smile on her face. I was absolutely
speechless. I was afraid to talk. I didn't know how to
approach him, what to say. I wanted to say only the
right things. I wanted his attention, his approval of my
body, his compliments, which I got. But it must have
been strange for him. I ran around like an excited little
kid, looking at his muscles, trying to talk to him—
which was difficult, since at the time I still didn't know
English well. But we had a beautiful communication
going without really having to say very much. For so
many years, Reg Park had been part of my life. Now I
could finally train with him, watch him. He was famous for certain muscles I didn't have—such as
calves, deltoids and abdominals. These are the major
muscles one needs to look really Herculean. That's
when I cut out the nonsense and started getting his
whole program down.

I went with Reg on the entire exhibition trip—to
Ireland, to Manchester and the different cities in England. We had the same kind of body, tall and wide
and huge, and this was appealing to a large audience.
At the first exhibition he introduced me to the audience, saying that as far as he was concerned I was the
next Mr. Universe. In a few years I was going to be the
greatest thing bodybuilding had ever seen.

I traveled with Reg Park for a week. I watched and
learned a lot. One inspiring thing was that his body
tuned in the same way mine did. We both liked the
heavy, heavy workouts with barbell sets and not as
much with dumbbells. It was fantastic having Reg Park
as a training partner, working with me, standing above
me to help if a weight was too heavy or I cramped up
from too many reps. I'm sure I wore him out during
the tour. There were so many things to talk about that

still seemed mysterious. Such as how different body-builders had to do different exercises for different body parts. According to Reg, the reason was bone structure. It was obvious, for example, that a guy with short legs had to do fewer squats before his legs would fill up much faster—which was why I should never squat with a short guy; my long legs required more squats, more weight.

Working with Reg Park for that short time helped more than anything to clear up the little confusions I had about the principles of other champions. I learned that you can't really say, "You must do this to get such and such a result." You have to try out certain things and find out what is best for your own body. I collected advice from Reg the whole time. I wrote it all down to take back to Munich and use as it seemed to serve me best. In the end, he promised he would invite me to South Africa the next year to do an exhibition with him. But he said it was contingent upon my winning Mr. Universe the coming year. He thought I would win for sure—if I worked hard.

Back at the gym, I trained almost totally according to Reg Park's principles and system: keep the exercises simple. There were certain moves he did that were different from mine and I adopted them. I knew that in the coming year I had to be supercritical. I had to analyze and work on my faults harder than ever before.

I discovered that taking measurements gave me both satisfaction and incentive. I measured my calves, arms and thighs regularly, and I'd be turned on if I saw I'd increased an eighth-inch or a half-inch. On a calendar I kept even fractional changes in measurements and weight. I had a photographer take pictures at least once a month. I studied each shot with a magnifying glass. I hung around people who were aware of physical shape and who could continually give me compliments. Suddenly I was up all the time. My confidence soared.

Meeting Reg Park helped me in a number of ways. One was to make me want to become a better person. There was a funny period I went through which began about the time I was nineteen. I'd become fully developed physically, weighing between 240 and 250 pounds. I'd begun to get a lot of notoriety and I started feeling superior to everyone. I think that when you're almost up to the top, but not quite there, it's easy to be carried away with what you imagine to be your own importance. I was pretty ego-oriented anyway. I already felt I was better than anyone else. I felt as if I were a Superman or something. That was my attitude: macho. I was strong and I walked the streets feeling and acting tough. If someone made the slightest remark or gave me trouble I would hit them over the head. I was aggressive and rude. I'd go into a beer hall where we ate dinner after training and start a fight for no reason at all.

It was a bad time. Now, looking back on it, I'm embarrassed. I was nothing more than a punk, a big bully throwing my weight around. I had fights almost every day. It might be in the train station with an Italian or a Greek. Or it might be in front of a girl, just to show off what kind of a man I was. I made a lot of trouble, got in scrapes with the police, drove crazily, collected handfuls of speeding tickets—they were all connected with my need to emphasize my masculinity, my superior size and strength. But when I'd finished my tour with Reg and built up the momentum of my training schedule for the Mr. Universe contest, I grew more and more satisfied with my progress and became aware of how good my body was, how good I was. Then gradually I could allow myself to admit how bad I was in other areas. The more I won, the more I started feeling like a human being again, just a normal guy. I became so content to work hard and drive myself to the top that the whole business of fighting and acting out the macho role went away. In the space of a month it was gone. I suddenly knew who I was. But in a way I think it was important for me to have gone through this period early, because I could look back, see how stupid the tough-guy stuff was, and not waste any more of my life.

The whole point of the tough-guy business was just to psych myself up, have another way of telling myself I was great. It was part of the winning trip. "I'm great, I'm the greatest." I was continuously trying to convince myself of it. In fact, I did it so well I forgot there was another life besides the life of a bodybuilder, besides my life. I was trying to prove something, because I was frustrated, because I was still not the best. I use a perfect example in the book *Pumping Iron*. When you have a BMW, which drives well although it's not a great car, you try to race with everybody to prove that it has speed. But when you have a Ferrari or a Lamborghini you *know* you can beat anybody on the street. You don't race any more. You start driving 55 on the freeway. Anybody can pass you and you know that if you step on the gas they're gone. You *know* how good you are, you don't have to prove it any more. It was the same for that period in my life. I wanted to think I was the greatest bodybuilder but I wasn't. Not yet. Not even in my mind. That's why I had to spend every minute trying to prove it.

My life changed in other areas. For the first time ever, I had a steady girl friend. It was the first stable relationship I'd had in a long time. It made training easier and calmed me down—I no longer had to prove through rudeness how much of a man I was.

Chapter Five

I knew I was a winner. I knew I was destined for great things. People will say that kind of thinking is totally immodest. I agree. Modesty is not a word that applies to me in any way—I hope it never will. But there are a number of things I had concluded about myself by that time—which was just prior to my second Mr. Universe contest. I'd formulated them in a simple list. I went down this list periodically and checked it off item by item.

Number One: I had the right chemistry. My bone structure was perfect—long legs, long arms, long torso. Plus, everything was in proportion. It fell together and flowed.

Number Two: I was learning to utilize both the good and bad points of my upbringing. Because of my strict parents, I was very disciplined. However, I didn't get certain things I needed as a child, and that, I think, finally made me hungry for achievement, for winning in other ways, for being the best, being recognized. If I'd gotten everything and been well-balanced, I wouldn't have had my drive. So, as a result of this negative element in my upbringing, I had a positive drive toward success and recognition.

Number Three: I started training in an area where there were no distractions; there was nothing else going on, and that gave me enough time to concentrate and find out what bodybuilding was really all about.

Number Four: I always had a positive attitude about going to the top. Never was there even the slightest doubt in my mind that I would make it. And this helped me keep training and trying. I was determined and constant. I never wanted to pause or stop training. I trained twelve months of the year, really hard, with no letup. Most of the bodybuilders didn't do that. I sacrificed a lot of things most bodybuilders didn't want to give up. I just didn't care, I wanted to win more than anything. And whatever it took to do it, I did.

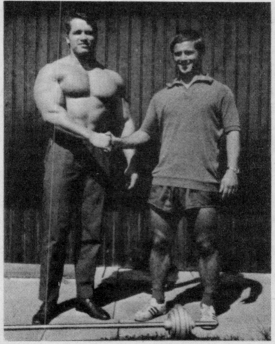

In Munich with Gerhard Mueller, the world's top soccer player, 1967

Number Five: I was honest with myself about what my body looked like and where I'd have to improve. As soon as I became aware of a weak point I went all out to eliminate it. For instance, in the beginning everybody said, "Arnold has no calves. Compared to his thighs or arms, his calves aren't developed at all." One look in the mirror told me they were right. I had to have better calves. I had to train my calves every day and twice as hard as any other muscle. That's what I did. And a year later I had calves. Then someone said to me, "Arnold, you don't have enough deltoids." So I trained my deltoids really hard. I developed my own exercise called the Arnold Press, a rotating exercise designed to work directly on the deltoid, which we will get into when we talk about training. All my energies, both psychic and physical, were focused on one thing: becoming Mr. Universe. It would not be a sure win— not at that point. I wasn't blind. I had weak points— glaring weak points—and I got to work on them. Many bodybuilders refuse to do this; they keep working on their strong points, which is more gratifying. But I didn't want the best arms or legs or chest. I wanted to be the best-built man in the world.

I knew I had what it took. Now I had to bring it all together. This took posing ability, showmanship. I had to be able to handle my body on the posing platform during prejudging. I refused to just imitate somebody else. I developed a posing routine that fit me and my body, my size and my style. I cut out magazine pictures of other bodybuilders posing. Sometimes I saved only the hands or the twist of the torso. I circled the part I liked. Sometimes the pictures were not of bodybuilders. I looked for models and dancers in poses I really liked, poses I thought I could do. I was trying for something distinctive, something strong and fluid and powerful and beautiful. When I put them all together, I had twenty poses. I went through them, arranging and modifying, working to tie one pose to another pose, until I had something that said *Arnold*.

I was a rough type, but with symmetry and elegance. I had to capture that style. Posing is an expression of you, it's a part of you. I was like a cat. My body was supple, smooth. I wanted a lot of movement in my posing routine, which was something I didn't see in many bodybuilders. I wanted to move like a cat, going gracefully from one pose to the next, making a lyrical sweep and then hitting it with power: *Boom!* Just like a cat when it jumps—making this beautiful, silent jump—then landing with a lot of noise and force. A cat kills, a big cat. And that's what I wanted to do.

I'd close my eyes and think about how I was going to look up there. I would visualize it and try to mold it together. Gradually I narrowed it down to the poses best suited for me, the strong, catlike poses, and I worked slowly at putting together a complete, flawless routine. I tried this routine at an exhibition and then asked people to criticize it. I insisted on hearing what they did not like. I got criticism from close friends, people who knew what I was up to and gave me honest feedback. I needed their criticism. I went home and worked on those weak points.

One word was constantly on my mind: *perfection*. I concentrated on remaining in a pose for a certain amount of time. It was important to hold it for a minute to get rid of the shaking and to let the muscles know how they should be flexed. I had my routine filmed, I ran it over and over. I watched myself. I analyzed my routine and criticized it. That's how I learned. I spent countless hours posing, more hours analyzing.

Posing is pure theater. I understand that and I love it. There are bodybuilders who put almost no time into posing. And, of course, they don't win.

I also spent time watching other guys pose, watching films of them, especially guys I was going to compete against, to determine their weak points, their strong points. Then, on the day of the contest, I could outpose them. I'd see where they did slow poses, and figure out how I could put in three poses for their one, and thus be able to show many more body parts to the judges. All of this together made me certain I'd win.

Each night before I went to sleep I thought, "The better you pose, Arnold, the more it will look as though you're really in charge of yourself. You can handle yourself. You are confident. You are good. The better poser you are, the fewer facial expressions you will make. Keep your face relaxed. Your face will show that you are a winner. You are a winner, Arnold." I wrote this down and put it where I would see it. I repeated it a dozen times a day.

Your mental attitude has a profound effect on the judges. When you compete, your whole attitude is important. You have to be proud, you have to stand proud, your moves should be full of pride. You can pose as a loser and you can pose as a winner. It's very hard to explain, but I always recognize the look when I see it. A typical loser will do a double biceps pose, for instance, and hide in it; he'll just hide behind his biceps. A winner will do a double biceps pose and really open up. With his motions, he says to the judges, "Look at these muscles!" That makes the difference. If he changes from one pose to another with a big sweeping motion, you know he's confident; and if he smiles, then you know he has it.

I had noticed one thing wrong with almost every one of my competitors. On the day of the competition they were concerned only about their own bodies—that *they* looked good. I always felt that was a mistake. If you have to worry about your body on the day of competition you're worrying about it a little bit too late. You should worry about your body during the year of training, and on the day of the competition you should worry about the other guys' bodies. Which means that you should think about them, analyze them, and act according to how they look and what they do. I prepared myself for it. If someone came up with one pose, I knew I could come back with another. I knew when to put my energy into serious posing in front of the judges; this is when you win or lose. Posing in front of the audience is less critical; it's a kind of ballet, where you basically go through the poses as a performer and there is no competition. Both times are serious—except that before the judges is when you'd better be making every move count.

One point in my favor was that my body has always been dramatic and spectacular, more than the average bodybuilder's. The main reason for this is a trait I share with Reg Park. I look very symmetrical when I stand relaxed, without the too-wide, squared shoulders and the arms that appear propped away from the ribs by a surplus of muscle that characterize most bodybuilders. I've never minded that my body doesn't look massive when I'm standing relaxed. It has always had a nice muscular look, but nothing freaky or unusual. I never tried to tense it up, to get musclebound. However, when I posed my whole physique would change radically. My body would open up like an accordion and my muscles would appear. Even in terms of measurements the difference was phenomenal. Hanging, my arm would measure 19 inches; when I flexed, it would balloon to 22 inches. The same thing was true of my chest. I could make my chest expand so dramatically it shocked people; they didn't know where it came from. My thighs always looked thin, too, but when I flexed they exploded. It was a direct result of working with more repetitions and less weight. Because if you always train with heavy weights you get to look like Franco Columbu; your muscles are always there. Then when you pose there's no real surprise. I don't want to knock that look. For myself, I prefer the more dramatic body, the showman's body.

I had won the Mr. Universe title in my mind. My imagination was primed, my body ready. I was working to create the greatest, most perfect body anybody had ever seen.

I had lists and charts of the things I needed to concentrate on pasted all over. I looked at them every day before I began working out. It became a twenty-four-hour-a-day job; I had to think about it all the time. I had to make it clear to my mind that now my calves were equally as important as my biceps. It took a while to get this idea firmly planted because for years my mind had been focused on biceps training as the most important element in bodybuilding.

I realized, too, that every muscle had to be separated from the next muscle. Some of the standard exercises didn't seem to work for me, so I had to develop exercises that would chisel into those muscle areas. Everything had to be separated, but it had to be tied together. What this meant in simple terms is that when you pose you ought to seem connected, but where your muscles connect there should be a split. For instance, the pectoral muscles and the deltoids should work together but there should be a definite groove where the two meet. Separation. Until that time, I had concentrated on mass and never bothered much about separation. I began to work to separate the muscles and get definition, which has to do with the configuration of the muscle itself.

I sought exercises that would burn off every gram of fat between the muscles. I went at it like a scientist. I had to find a way to separate the deltoid from the trapezius. I developed an upward rowing exercise which I did on the beach with heavy weights. Then I came up with an exercise to separate the pectorals from the deltoid, which I called front raises with dumbbells. I did dips to separate the pectorals from the abdominals.

My calves were still weak. I started training them before I did the rest of my workout, so I could put more weight on the machine and really blast them. If I couldn't get enought weight on the machine, I got the biggest guy in the gym to sit on top of it. I began flexing my thighs, flexing my calves. I did a lot of tensing after each workout, employing it as a kind of super-isometrics. I posed before a morror constantly. I spent hours lying in the sun to burn off the fat tissue just under the skin.

Now every time I did an exhibition people would say, "I can't believe the improvement you've made, Arnold. You're getting more definition. All of a sudden you don't look so rough any more. More quality is coming out." I got feedback on those changes and I dug it. I could tense my legs now and see that my calves had come in. This gave me even greater confidence and drive. I recorded my progress on the charts I'd been keeping. And I pushed myself harder.

The reason for the acceleration in the final few weeks was that I had heard rumors of a new rival. Dennis Tinnerino had just won Mr. America and was already spoken of in some circles as the new Mr. Universe. I got his pictures and checked them: he looked fantastic. Still, he didn't have great arms, and I felt I had a better back and chest. But I recognized that his legs were better developed than mine. I had worked hard, but it's impossible to transform legs very much in a single year. I felt I could almost equal him in legs, and in the other areas I felt I had him—hands down.

I compared myself with Tinnerino's pictures—although photographs are very deceiving. I was even more critical of myself than ever. I was taping my measurements and weighing myself every few days now. I was cutting myself down for the competition. Two weeks before the contest I did an exhibition in Wales. People told me I looked fantastic. But they had magazines with cover photographs of Dennis Tinnerino, and they were skeptical of my chances. They kept saying, "This is the guy you have to beat, Arnold. Look at how cut he is, look at his definition." Tinnerino was the contender. I didn't know if Chet Yorton was coming back or not, but it didn't matter because now I could beat him easily. Dennis Tinnerino was obviously my biggest threat.

When I returned to London from Wales, I trained one afternoon with Ricky Wayne. He was living in London and editing the English version of *Muscle Builder* magazine. He shook his head and said Tinnerino was so cut up, so incredible, that I didn't have a chance. I felt the sting of Ricky's words. He saw it and shrugged. That's the way it was. I refused to believe it. Ricky went on to compound it with Tinnerino's statistics. Measurements have always been exaggerated in muscle magazines, so I wasn't worried about the measurements. But I could see from the photographs that Tinnerino was finished. He was stunning.

"Okay," I thought, "he looks like a winner but I'm going to beat him anyway." I went back to Munich with less than two weeks until contest time. I trained harder than ever. I even went to the gym the morning of the day before the contest and put in three grueling hours. Then I caught a flight to London. I landed at midnight and decided not to go to bed. I was so busy psyching myself up for the contest, I couldn't have slept anyway. Besides, I felt that staying up all night would burn off an extra few calories around my waist.

At six the next morning I took the elevator down to the street. Already a crowd of bodybuilders was standing in front of the Royal Hotel. They'd probably all been too nervous to sleep, too.

Tinnerino had come over from America with his manager, Leo Stern. Stern had taken him away from the whole scene, to create suspense, to keep people from seeing him before the contest.

My friend Wag Bennett, who was one of the judges, met me that morning. He was helping me, giving me instructions, psyching me up. He had seen Tinnerino and agreed it would be close. I had brought a photographer friend with me, Albert Busek, and I sent him out as a spy to locate Tinnerino and see how he looked. Obviously, I was uneasy. Albert persuaded Leo Stern to let him in to take some pictures of Tinnerino. When he returned I could see he'd been impressed. "Arnold," he said, almost as if he wished he didn't have to tell me, "Tinnerino *is* incredible."

Finally that morning at the prejudging I saw Tinnerino myself. He had come down to watch the short and medium men compete. We talked briefly. But it was one of those situations where we were trying to psych each other out. He asked me how I was and I said, "Fantastic!" I leaned closer. "It's the kind of day when you know you're going to win." I smiled and let my body open out slowly. I felt cocky. But I meant it. I was going to beat him.

The prejudging of the tall men's class was in the afternoon at one o'clock. I went up to take a nap at lunchtime and didn't wake up until exactly one o'clock, when I heard Albert pounding on my door. He was yelling at me, saying I was going to be disqualified if I wasn't onstage in ten minutes. I woke up in a daze, grabbed my posing trunks, and ran downstairs—the lineup was standing there, ready, waiting. I ran by, and it was kind of great. I mean there they all were, all pumped up, this awesome proliferation of muscles, and I was coming in cold and they knew it. I took a look at Dennis Tinnerino and I wasn't all that impressed. He was in shape, he was cut, but he could have been bigger and better. That's what I thought.

I changed clothes quickly, smoothed on a little oil, and hurried back to the platform. I didn't have time to pump up at all. But I had begun to get that feeling of magnificence I always have at a contest. I took a place in line right next to Tinnerino. He was the man to beat. I didn't want the judges to make any mistakes because they couldn't compare us. I heard all kinds of noise, everybody was talking about us. There was so much talking going on, the judges stopped calling poses. It was a strange moment. I remember checking out the lineup, getting my sights set on the competition. It was a cluster of bodies that might have been polished brass, skin burnished with oil until it shone in the stage light. Finally they quieted the people down and started calling for poses again. After the lineup came the individual posing. It was run off according to height, the shorter ones first. I was tallest, so I was last, after Tinnerino. That meant I would be the final attraction. Perfect.

I watched every move Tinnerino made. He posed and got a lot of applause. He was very professional; he had spent time on all the details—trunks, hairstyle, everything. But I knew I could upstage him. Tall, easy, confident, I moved like a cat onto the posing platform. I felt good. My body was pumped and tight, blood surging out to every capillary. I just felt that there was no way Tinnerino could beat me. And I generated that onstage.

When I hit my first arm pose the place fell apart; everybody started roaring. I swept into a back pose and the same thing happened. I limited my routine to ten poses (normally I'd do fifteen to twenty poses). I used only my best shots and left out anything I thought had even the slightest weak point. I did a side-back-down position, changed to a side chest shot, another back pose, a straight-on back shot, then finished with a side biceps pose. I had people screaming and whistling and hollering. I came back to the front for another double biceps pose. Then I finished off with the Most Muscular pose. Everybody started applauding and applauding and going crazy. Usually at the prejudging applause is not allowed because it might influence the judges. But the people couldn't hold themselves back. This was my pump-up. Blood was rushing to every single area of my body. I didn't need to do anything physical any more to pump up.

The time came for the pose-off. After the individual posing, the judges called out the top six guys; they stand you in a line and call out the poses you are to do. They asked for a double biceps pose. I knew I had everyone beat there. Then a lat spread. I felt good with that one. Next they asked for a side chest pose. I knew I had the best chest. Then they asked for abdominals. Dennis Tinnerino had me in the abdominals; he had tight, quilted abdominals. He also beat me on calves. Then we were allowed to do our favorite poses. And all my rehearsing really helped me. I stood right next to Tinnerino and watched him constantly out of the corner of my eye. When he showed his abs or thighs, I hit a biceps pose; when he twisted to flex his calves, I drew myself up in a dramatic side-chest-back pose. I wiped everybody, including Tinnerino, off the stage. I got the best reaction—it was the first time I remember people really screaming, "Arnold! Arnold!"

The judges came over afterward and complimented me. Without being too obvious, they gave me a great deal of special attention. Some judges felt I was better in every single muscle. From this, I was almost certain I'd won. Still, Tinnerino had me in certain areas. But I had a better posing routine, a better all-around presentation. The winner would not be announced until the next day, at the actual show. That meant waiting. People kept coming up and telling me I was the most sensational thing they'd ever seen. I liked hearing that, of course. But it was the judges' decision that counted, and I was waiting for the show the next evening.

Bodybuilders and fans hung around me that whole day. Everybody already assumed I was the winner. They started treating me as Mr. Universe. That was one of the great experiences of my life. But it was unsettling too. I still didn't know for sure whether or not I was the winner. I went to my room. But I couldn't stay in. I took the elevator down to the lobby of the hotel. Again, people congratulated me. "Don't worry, Arnold, you've got it." All I could do was wait and not let on that not a single cell in my body would accept second place. I walked around, let people compliment me, and listened to the comments they thought I couldn't hear. I confess I loved it when they called me a monster. "Look," they'd hiss. "It's Arnold. He's an animal."

The next night, for the final show when the winners would be announced and from them the Mr. Universe selected, I made sure I was not caught sleeping. Backstage, the atmosphere was intensely theatrical. I found the dressing room for the tall men's class. I started pumping up half an hour before the show, working especially on all the things I thought were my weak points. I did chin-ups on water pipes—the first one was hot and I burned my hands. I did towel-pulls, handstand push-ups, regular push-ups, dips between chairs, curls with towels, using any kind of a resistance movement I could for a pump. I got somebody to press down on my arms so I could do lateral raises, and force blood into the area of the deltoids, just to get the blood circulating. I did calf raises with one leg, sissy squats, just going down partway with my back straight, to put a little blood in the frontal thigh—I didn't want to pump the thigh too much, otherwise I'd lose it again before I went onstage.

We were like gladiators. There was oil all over the place; people were speaking different languages; French, English, Portuguese, German, Arabic. Across the room somebody did a stretching exercise and nearly ripped out a water pipe. I stepped across the room and bent it back in place, as though I were the only one strong enough to do it. I knew guys were watching me. I was flexing. I was being domineering, the winner. Then one of the officials stuck his head in the doorway and yelled, "Okay, tall men out! Stand out in line."

"All right, Arnold," I said to myself. "This is it."

For some reason, waiting there beside the folds of velour curtain in the old theater, I found myself thinking back to my first contest—Mr. Europe Junior. I'd gone to Stuttgart with no posing experience, AWOL from the Army, wearing one of their bad haircuts, in borrowed posing trunks, and I'd won. It struck me how far I'd come in such a short time. . . .

As soon as I began posing I got thundering applause from the British audience. What I was doing now was mostly for exhibition and my routine became ballet. I had to come back for an encore. I was the only guy who had to pose a second time. They announced the height class winners. I won in the tall men, which automatically made me the winner, because I knew I had only had to beat Dennis Tinnerino. And I'd done that.

All the height class winners were standing there, the short, medium and tall winners. The crowd was going crazy. Again they were yelling, "Arnold! Arnold!" I felt their energy, their enthusiasm running through my body like this fantastic pump. It seemed my body just grew and grew. Finally the announcer got the crowd quieted down enough so he could announce third place, second place and the winner, Mr. Universe 1967.

"Arnold Schwarzenegger—"

I heard my name and stepped up on the platform. The applause was like thunder roaring through the auditorium. People were shouting and clamoring. I looked at the lineup of bodybuilders and said to myself, "My god, I did it. I beat them all." It was the first time in a year I had allowed myself to acknowledge how good they looked. There were ninety bodybuilders there from all over the world. And I had beaten

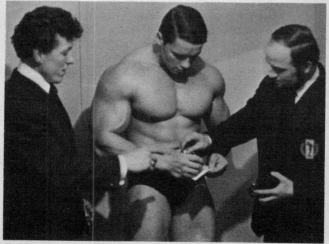

At nineteen years old

them all. A million things went through my mind at that moment. It's like when you have an accident or when you're just about to fall. A whole lifetime goes through your mind in a single second. You picture yourself being dead, or you imagine what might happen to your family.

After they announced the winners it took a few minutes to hand out the trophies. I looked out at the audience. They were screaming, flashbulbs were going off, I was caught up in the strange, unreal splendor of it. I thought, This is what you have been training for, this moment. There was just no way I could take it all in. It was like confronting something impossible to lift. I tried to come down, to realize what it meant. "What is happening right now, now," I told myself, "is the most important moment in your life." It was what I had meant when I made up my mind at the age of ten to be the greatest person in one field. I was twenty years old and I was already the greatest and the best.

I repeated it over to myself: Arnold Schwarzenegger, Mr. Universe 1967.

Chapter Six

Sunday morning I went downstairs for breakfast. It was a scene out of a Marx Brothers film. In the dining room I saw at least fifty bodybuilders wearing their special jackets with wide padded shoulders. Some guys were having ten eggs, some guys two steaks, some guys only two eggs because they were on a diet. One guy was eating fifteen pieces of toast. As soon as I walked in, everybody started waving at me. They crowded around my table. They were very affectionate, especially the Arabs. They came over and kissed me and hugged me. They were happy for my success. Someone leaned across the table and said, "Okay, Arnold, the next one is Sergio Oliva."

"What?"

"No," said someone else, "the next one is Bill Pearl."

They mentioned all the great names of the bodybuilding world who were still out there in front of me, guys I still had to beat. Which totally blew my mind. I was Mr. Universe, but I wasn't. They had to explain it to me. I *was* Mr. Universe, but a few months before there'd been another Mr. Universe contest, run by the IFBB, another bodybuilding federation. The winner of that had been Sergio Oliva, a black bodybuilder from Cuba. The truth was, there were three Mr. Universes. One was Bill Pearl, who had won the NABBA professional Mr. Universe title, while I'd won the NABBA

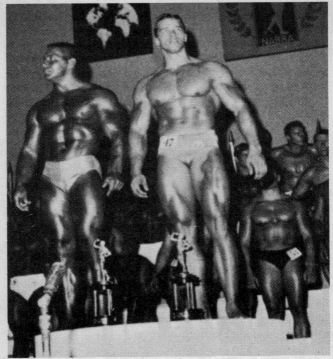

Posing with Bill Pearl after winning my first Mr. Universe contest, 1967

amateur Mr. Universe title. There was the IFBB Mr. Universe, Sergio Oliva. (There are two different international bodybuilding federations, the National Amateur Bodybuilding Association and the IFBB, which is the International Federation of Bodybuilding. Both have Mr. Universe contests.) Then, too, there was Ricky Wayne, who had just won the Mr. World contest in New York. Sergio Oliva had also won the Mr. Olympia contest.

At least I knew this much: I was now one of the four top bodybuilders in the world. Which was an accomplishment. But there were three other guys out there I had to beat to let everybody know I was indisputably the best. I had achieved one goal, which was winning a Mr. Universe title. But I had to go on. Otherwise I wouldn't be satisfied. Take the Olympics, for example. The guy who wins the Olympic medal has done a great thing, but he's not the best in the world. You're only best when you beat all the competition. Because some guy might have an injury, or some guy couldn't make it to the meet—say he overslept (I knew that could happen) and he couldn't make it, as with the runner who missed the 100 yard sprint in 1972. There are certain things you can win and still not be sure you are the best. So if it's important for you to be the best and not just the winner, and it was for me, then you go on. That was my next challenge, to be the best, the ultimate winner. I vowed to keep going on and on and on until everybody in the world said, "Yes, it's him. It's Arnold, he's the best."

But that Sunday morning I was inundated with questions. "How do you train?" "Why is your chest so big?" "Why won't mine grow?" "Why are your biceps so huge?" "How did you improve your thighs so much in one year, Arnold?"

I didn't see Dennis Tinnerino until a few days later. He was known to be a playboy. He always had girls around him. That seemed to be one of his main concerns—being there, having a good time, and being crazy. A week after the Mr. Universe contest we did an exhibition together for Wag Bennett. I tried to talk to him then. My English was much better than it had been the previous year, but I still found it hard to have a conversation with him. He was very friendly to me. He must have been disappointed. The press had built him up as a sure winner. But he didn't show any signs that he thought the judging had been unfair. He came to me before the exhibition, said I looked fantastic, that I had deserved to win. I asked Tinnerino what I should do to improve. "Keep working on your calves,

Arnold," he said. He turned his right leg and flexed. He had really gorgeous calves which popped out like small melons.

One disappointing note was struck when I called my parents and told them I was Mr. Universe. They seemed excited to hear from me, but I felt that if it had been through the local Graz paper saying I had just completed my college degree, it would have meant more to them. After I hung up the phone I felt depressed. I told myself it was because they couldn't relate to a world championship in bodybuilding. Because they had never seen anything like it.

In a way I cared that they didn't understand it. I felt they ought to have at least realized what it meant to me. They knew how hard I had worked for it. I tried to put it out of my mind, but it wasn't easy. I think you're always doing things for the approval of your parents. I think I understood them, their shortcomings, better than they understood me. I convinced myself I should forget it. I was away from home anyway, so I started looking for the approval of the other people.

A few weeks after the Mr. Universe contest I did an exhibition in Stuttgart and my father came to watch me. He was excited about the fact that I got a lot of applause. That hit home for him. I don't think it occurred to him that they cheered and applauded because I was Mr. Universe, that they liked my body, which was one of the best-developed bodies in the world—even then. He knew there were 2,000 people who had come to see me pose. But that's as much as he understood of it. And my mother even less—until much later, when she saw me win the Mr. Olympia contest in 1972.

A short time after the contest I received an invitation from Reg Park asking me to come to South Africa, stay at his house, and do the exhibition he had promised. I was in my glory. My friends were astounded. I trained as vigorously in preparation for this exhibition as I had for any contest I had ever participated in. I don't know how many years I'd dreamed about being like Reg Park; then, all of a sudden, I was really almost like him. People remarked on it. They said we shared that rugged, heroic quality.

I stayed with Reg in Johannesburg. He had a beautiful sprawling single-story house with an Olympic-size pool in front, the whole thing surrounded by a rose garden and acres of flowers and trees. The house itself was filled with antiques from all over the world. It had an aura about it: it was the house of a star. That quality was unmistakable. In the dining room, for instance, you pressed a button and servants appeared.

At first I felt out of place, but before long my discomfort disappeared. Reg and his wife, Maryanne, treated me as if I were their son. They included me in everything they did; they took me to parties, films, dinners. Being with them opened my mind to what was possible for me aside from endless days taken up totally with training. I could have a gorgeous house, businesses, a family, a good life. Being with them, I

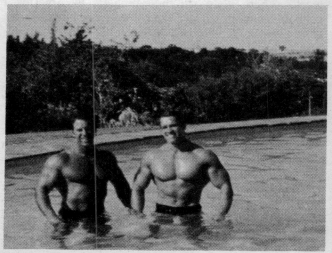

With Reg Park at his home in South Africa

felt fulfilled. It was a unique experience for me to see
Reg at home, to be with him that long, and to get so
much attention from him.

It wasn't all praise. I asked him for criticism and I
got it. He, too, singled out my calves. He said he'd had
the same problem, but he had overcome it. I soon
learned why. I watched him do his calf workouts and
he put me to shame. I was putting small weights on the
machine. He stepped over, ran it up to 800 pounds,
and did twelve reps. I knew then that as relentlessly as
I'd trained, I needed to work even harder if I wanted to
reach the plateau he was on.

When I arrived back in Munich, more people enrolled in my gymnasium. Membership increased to
about 400. Money started coming in. Money meant
freedom; that in turn meant time to train. So everything began going well.

I had discovered that winning the Mr. Universe contest doesn't make you the best bodybuilder in the
world. There were still bodybuilders in America I
probably couldn't beat. This was a big blow. There
were some guys who had won the Mr. Universe contest two and three times. I figured I had to compete
two or three more times before I would have finally
conquered everybody.

I set myself a schedule to train straight through the
entire year again. I began blasting my body in the gym,
going early in the morning, staying late at night, doing
some ferocious work. I had no trouble getting training
partners. Every bodybuilder in Munich wanted to train
with Arnold. They thought I knew some secret. We
got into forced reps, real torture routines where we
pushed ourselves beyond the point of pain. We ate
enormous meals. After each workout we would go to
the beer hall and devour a whole chicken each and
mugs of beer. That was our dinner. In the actual training routines I was trying to be more creative than I'd
ever been, putting my imagination into play in an at-

tempt to figure out how I could go beyond everyone else. If someone could get a 21-inch arm, I would blow mine up to 22 inches.

Arnold, I asked myself over and over, "What can you do to be special and different?"

I finally arrived at the idea of shocking the muscles. If you do ten sets of bench presses or any other exercise regularly for a year, the muscles gradually get used to ten sets of bench presses and the growth slows down. So once a week I took a training partner and drove out into the country with the weights. We limited ourselves to one exercise for a particular body part. I remember for the first day we carried 250 pounds out into the forest and did squats for three hours straight. I began by doing twenty repetitions with 250 pounds; then my partner did whatever he could. Then it was my turn again. We ended up doing something like fifty-five sets of squats each. The last hour seemed endless. But it worked. Our thighs pumped up like balloons. That first day we gave our thigh muscles such a shock that we couldn't walk right for a week. We barely could crawl. Our legs had never experienced anything as tough as those fifty-five sets. And each of us put something like an eighth or a quarter of an inch on our thighs; they just blew up, they had no chance to survive except to grow.

We made it a regular thing. We brought girls out there to cook. We made a fire outdoors and turned the whole thing into a little contest. We worked hard but we had a good time. After the muscle-shocking sessions we drank wine and beer and got drunk and carried on like the old-time weight lifters back in the 1800s or early 1900s. Sometimes it became pure insanity. We'd grab up the weights again, but we were weaker because of the beer, and the weights would fall back over our heads. Or we'd get them down on our chests and wouldn't be able to press them on up from there and someone would have to lift them off for us. It was a great time. We cooked shish kebab, sat around the fire, and made love. We got into this trip that we were gladiators, male animals. We swam naked out in nature, had all this food, wine and women; we ate like animals and acted like animals. We got off on it so much it became a weekly routine—eating fresh meat and drinking wine and exercising.

It's important that you like what you do, and we loved it. We had fun, but we also did astonishing workouts. We did tortuous workouts in the fresh air. We challenged each other. We experienced a lot of pain. We'd be in the middle of a squat and just cramp up. We'd roll on the ground and try to massage it out. That was the first time I knew pain could become pleasure. We were benefiting from pain. We were breaking through the pain barrier and shocking the muscle. We looked at this pain as a positive thing, because we grew.

It was a fantastic feeling to gain size from pain. All of a sudden I was looking forward to it as something pleasurable. The whole idea of pain became a pleasure trip. I couldn't tell anybody about it then, because I knew they would say I was a weirdo, a masochist. Which wasn't true, I had just converted the pain into pleasure—not for its own sake but because it meant growing. We bragged to each other about how much it hurt.

Every weekend we would do the same thing, with bench presses, rowing, or flyes, bombing our bodies, giving them something different from the usual everyday routine. The theory was this: surprise the body. Don't always do what it expects. This was a new way of promoting muscle growth. I saw it having amazing results on me and I started to preach this as a method for bodybuilding.

I learned about things like the split routine, the shock method, breaking through the pain barrier, all for practical reasons: I wanted bigger, better muscles. None of this came from other bodybuilders. They were all my own ideas, completely original methods, designed by me for my body. I believe the same thing has been done by other great bodybuilders, and anyone who ever wanted to go beyond the established limits in any field. Your first concern must be yourself. You have to invent the means to take you over the top. For instance, the first three years I was training, I found that when I was doing a dumbbell curl with my wrist straight I felt it in my biceps. However, when I did the curl and turned my wrist I felt it more intensely; I felt it reaching into a particular area of the elbow that hadn't been affected before. I asked why I should feel it there, and my doctor friend came up with the answer that the biceps' job is not only to lift the forearm up to flex but also to turn the wrist. If the biceps' job is to turn the wrist, I wondered why I shouldn't make it more difficult to turn the dumbbell. So I made one side of my dumbbells heavier, throwing them out of balance, and instantly I could feel what it did for my biceps. I was sore all the time. These were ideas I never found in books and magazines. I wanted to grow so fast and be so special I just accepted that I would have to invent new ways of working on the muscles.

Life in Munich was as crazy as ever. We worked hard, but we had fun. There was a lot of beer drinking, partying. It was a happy, beautiful time. I was young and becoming famous. In Munich itself I was looked upon as a freak celebrity, Arnold the muscleman. But I was proud of my achievements and I was letting it be known that this was only the beginning. Not many people were willing to argue with me. I saw myself as being able to help bodybuilding transcend its unfortunate reputation as an oddball sport.

Every year, in the spring, a stone-lifting contest is held in Munich. This has been going on for decades and has a lot of prestige in sporting circles. You stand on two footrests that look like chairs and pull the stone up between your legs by a metal handle. The stone

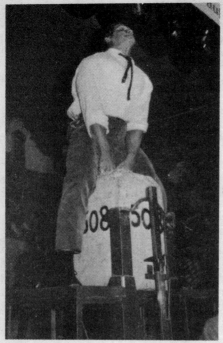

Stonelifting in Munich,
1967

weighs approximately 508 German pounds (about 560
English pounds). An electric scale on the wall of the
auditorium shows how many centimeters you lift the
stone. You do it cold; there's no warming up. You just
lift it up as far as you can. That year I entered the
contest, broke the existing record, and won. The press
picked it up and wrote that Mr. Universe was the
strongest man in Germany—which may or may not
have been true, but it was good for bodybuilding. At
that time, along with all the other misconceptions
about the sport, people still thought bodybuilders had
muscles but didn't have any power, just big useless
muscles.

I had met Franco Columbu at one of the weight-lifting contests that fall. For his size, he was one of the strongest men I'd ever seen. We became friends and started working out together. I liked training with Franco because he was so powerful. He was hardly a perfect specimen. When I first met him he seemed about as far from a Mr. Universe candidate as possible. He had a strange split in his chest; he was bow-legged; there were absolutely no visible signs of a champion in him. But I inspired him enough to want to be a muscleman, a champion with a beautiful physique, not just a powerlifting champion. I did it because of something I'd seen in Franco, which was his incredible willpower. He'd do squats with 300 pounds or 400 pounds, making as many as eight repetitions. Then one day he couldn't even get them up once. I had to help him. I couldn't believe it. Franco was always better at powerlifting than I was. Now I saw my chance to beat him. I said, "I bet you twenty marks I can get more reps than you."

"All right, Arnold." He looked at me for a moment. He lifted the bar off the squat rack and did ten smooth, sure repetitions.

His sudden comeback went churning around in my head for days. Why had Franco changed so rapidly? Obviously, in five minutes his body could not have changed. The only thing that had changed was his mind. Franco had set his immediate goal: "I want to beat Arnold. The guys are around. My ego is in jeopardy. I have to beat him now. Twenty marks, that's a nice meal." He made up these little goals. And he told himself he had to do ten repetitions. And he did. He went up and down like a piston. He could have done two more repetitions easily.

When I saw this in Franco, I knew he could go all the way. I knew too that he was the training partner who could whether the ferocious workouts necessary in the coming year. There grew up between us a perfect partnership. Franco saw me working and he started growing. I talked him into competing. He won a fourth-place trophy, then third-place and second-place trophies. In 1968 he won his height class in the Mr. Europe contest. That same year, he won second in his height class in the Mr. Universe contest. That gave him enough confidence to be a serious bodybuilder, to dedicate his life to it. Some phenomenal things happened to him because of his positive attitude. He too got obsessed with the idea of being the best.

The point is, I was learning more and more about the mind, about the power it has over the body. It meant having complete communication with the muscles, always feeling what was happening to my muscles the day after a workout. The most important thing is that my mind was always in touch with my body; I felt my muscles continuously; I always took an inventory before working out. I flexed my muscles and got in touch. That not only helped me train; it was like meditating. I locked my mind into my muscle during training, as if I'd transplanted my mind into the tissue itself. By just thinking about it, I could actually send blood into a muscle.

I formalized it by regularly making an inventory. How does my body feel now? I would ask myself. How does my chest feel? What did I get out of this press behind the neck, doing ten repetitions instead of five repetitions? How are my triceps? It doesn't do any good to go through training like a blind man, to just go through the motions. Motions mean nothing. You have to realize what is happening to you. You have to want results.

Bodybuilders hung on to me like fleas, because they thought if they did the same exercises I did they would get the same kind of muscles. But I watched them fall away with absolutely no results except exhaustion. They weren't mentally prepared for intensive championship training; they weren't thinking about it. I knew the secret: Concentrate while you're training. Do not allow other thoughts to enter your mind.

It became part of my routine that year to start out every day with total concentration. The way I did it was to play out exactly what I was going to use, how I was going to pull my muscles, and how I would feel it. I programmed myself. I saw myself doing it; I imagined how I would feel it. I was thoroughly, totally into it mentally. I did not waver at all.

When I went to the gym I got rid of every alien thought in my mind. I tuned in to my body as though it were a musical instrument I was about to play. In the dressing room I would start thinking about training, about every body part, what I was going to do, how I was going to pump up. I would concentrate on procedure and results until my everyday problems went floating away. I knew that if I went in there concerned about bills or girls and let myself think about those things while doing bench presses, I'd made only marginal progress. I'd seen guys reading the newspaper between sets day after day, and they always looked bad. Some of them had been going through the motions of training for years, and you couldn't tell that they had ever picked up a weight. It had been nothing more than some heartless pantomime.

During the first three years, in Austria, I had concentrated on my muscles naturally. I knew no other way. I grew up in a town where there were no distractions, and I had no personal problems. But Munich was different. Life there was fast. Opportunities cropped up continuously. I went out on dates and I traveled a great deal. And I soon discovered that if I allowed them to, other things could take my concentration away from bodybuilding. When I caught myself getting too involved thinking about my dates I saw how much it hurt my training. I'd fail to do bench presses with a strong groove, and the weight would seem heavier.

It was then I started seriously analyzing what happens to the body when the mind is tuned in, how important a positive attitude is. I questioned myself: Why you, Arnold? How did you win Mr. Universe after only five years of training? Other people asked me the same question. I began looking at the difference between me and other bodybuilders. The biggest difference was that most bodybuilders did not think *I'm going to be a winner.*They never allowed themselves to think in those terms. I would hear them complaining while they were training, "Oh, no, not another set!" The negative impulses around a gym can be incredible. Most of the people I observed couldn't make astonishing advances because they never had faith in themselves. They had a hazy picture of what they wanted to look like someday, but they doubted they could realize it. That destroyed them. It's always been my belief that if you're training for nothing, you're wasting your effort. Ultimately, they didn't put out the kind of effort I did because they didn't feel they had a chance to make it. And of course, starting with that premise, they didn't.

My analysis didn't stop with bodybuilding. I talked to weightlifting champions and they told me the same thing: it's in the mind. I knew from my own experience lifting weights that you stand in front of the bar and talk to it; you have to communicate with the bar: "You son-of-a-bitch, I'm going to rip you off my chest, I'm going to throw you over my head, I don't care how much you weigh. I'm the man who's going to take you out. I'm going to be the master of you." You talk yourself into it. You tell yourself you are going to be the hero. And you picture yourself completing the lift before you even touch the weights. With weight lifters, the psyching-up process can be endless. That's why the tournament officials introduced the rule that a man is allowed only three minutes' pause from one lift to the next. Given the chance, some guys would stand there for an hour preparing their minds for some giant press. But that's the way these lifters master weight. If they have lifted it mentally, they will undoubtedly lift it physically. There's no two ways about it, because they've done all the training, their bodies are ready; now it's only the mind. The mind must carry through.

If a man stands there and thinks for one-tenth of a second, "Maybe I can't lift it," it's gone. He will not make the lift. Proof of my point is that for years weight lifters could not lift more than 500 pounds. Nobody could. They did 499½ but never 500. The reason was this supposedly insurmountable mental barrier that had existed for years. They stood in front of the weight thinking, "No one has ever lifted 500 pounds. Why should I be the one?" Then in 1970 Alexiev of Russia lifted 501 pounds. He broke the barrier. A month after that, three or four guys lifted 500 pounds. Why? They believed it was possible. Reddig from Belgium lifted over 500 pounds. An American, Ken Pentera, went over 500. A month later another Russian lifted over 500. Now it's up to 564 pounds. The body didn't change. How could the body change that much in ten years? It was the same body. But the mind was different. Mentally it's possible to break records. Once you understand that, you can do it.

The year 1968 was intense. I worked out two and three hours at a stretch twice a day. I had enrolled in business school, trying to supplement the courses I'd had in high school. If I wasn't training or taking care of the gym, I was in class or studying. The energy and momentum around me was unbelievable. I was insatiable, unstoppable. My friends were shaking their heads. "Arnold," they'd say, "you're crazy. You're going to burn yourself out. Slow down." I laughed at them and pushed myself that much harder.

I arrived at the contest in London in that same spirit. I was every inch the winner. I knew that. I walked as though I already had the title won, as though there was no question that I would win and that the second-place man would be trailing points behind me. I was so huge and confident. And naturally I won. It could not have been otherwise.

Winning my second Mr. Universe title, the Mr. Universe Professional (NABBA), opened up a whole new world for me. Joe Weider, publisher of *Muscle Builder and Mr. America* magazines and owner of the various Weider Enterprises, which serve the bodybuilding world, got in touch with me. He asked if I'd come to America to compete in the IFBB Mr. Universe contest in Miami, Florida, because I'd told him over the phone that I was interested. He said that then we could discuss the possibility of my remaining in America for a few months, training in California.

Everything seemed to be happening right. My biggest dream had always been to go to America and train with the American bodybuilders. I wanted to learn

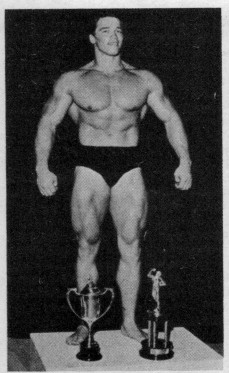

Mr. Universe for the second time, at twenty-one, 1968

from them, to get more information and—ultimately—to beat them. One thing I knew very little about at the time was the nutrition and drugs involved in body-building. Americans had been the experts in scientific bodybuilding for a long time. It was a fact that up until then America had produced most of the best bodybuilders in the world. Since the percentage had been so high, I thought there must be a reason. Perhaps it was knowledge, or better food, or better drugs. If not these things, maybe it was just being surrounded by the best bodybuilders—as in Gold's Gym. Positive thinking can be contagious. Being surrounded by winners helps you develop into a winner. Whatever it was, I was convinced that the answers were in America.

I arrived in Florida still totally confident. I felt I was ready. I'd just won in London and the heat of victory was in my blood. At the contest, people immediately crowded around to have a look at my body. The Americans had never seen me and they were amazed by my size.

When I went out to pose there was a strange silence, which puzzled me; I realized people were studying me. I gave them the biceps. Someone gasped. I could feel the crowd on the edges of their seats. It hit me then that this was America. I rose up and expanded every muscle fiber in my body. The crowd sensed it and cheered. I heard Americans shouting "Arnold!" I felt fantastic.

It wasn't until the pose-off that I realized how close a contest it was. There were guys here I'd never seen before. Frank Zane, in the medium class, had unbe-lievable cuts and an elegant posing routine. He posed gracefully, like a matador, like a dancer. His body seemed to have been tooled down with the chisels and gouges a sculptor would use on mahogany. The an-nouncer called out my name for second place. I was stunned. Frank Zane had won the IFBB Mr. Universe.

I came in second, on grounds that I was not defined enough, not perfectly developed. I was just the big-gest, not the best.

That did a little number on my mind. I went away
from the auditorium overwhelmed, crushed. I remember the words that kept going through my head: "I'm
away from home, in this strange city, in America, and
I'm a loser. . . ." I cried all night because of it. I had
disappointed all my friends, everybody, especially myself. It was awful. I felt it was the end of the world.

But I've always been resilient. A day later I had
gotten myself together. I'm going to pay them back, I
thought. I'm going to show them who is really the best.

I would train in America. I would use their food and
their knowledge and work it against them. I would
make it in America too.

Chapter Seven

I worked out an agreement with Joe Weider to spend one year in America. I would keep the gymnasium in Munich, have someone run it, and decide later if I wanted to stay or not. My desire, which I knew I could accomplish, was to train one whole year and beat everybody in America. My part of the agreement was to make available to Weider information about how I trained. He agreed to provide an apartment, a car, and to pay me a weekly salary in exchange for my information and being able to use photographs of me in his magazine. But the main thing I had was time, the freedom to stay and train four or five hours a day and compete in next year's IFBB Mr. Universe contest in New York.

Weider was seriously interested in me. I had come up extremely fast. At twenty-one, I weighed 250 pounds and had bigger measurements than any bodybuilder in the business. He knew I wanted to be the best and he saw the potential in me. It was good for both of us.

I was excited. For as long as I had been involved in bodybuilding, I'd been aware of Joe Weider. I had read *Muscle Builder* and *Mr. America* magazines. I knew about his barbells, food supplements and the various other products he sold for the sport. He had contacted me because I could be useful to him. I accepted that. But I knew he could be useful to me.

There were still a number of important goals before me, and this man could help me realize them.

I found out right away that Joe had two personalities. The warm, beautiful, human Joe Weider in his private life, and the shrewd businessman at the office.

I admire both sides of the man. Business fascinates me. I get caught up in the whole idea that it's a game to make money and to make money make more money. Joe Weider is a wizard at it, and I liked being able to watch him operate. But I especially liked the humanistic side of Weider. When he comes to my parties or when we go out to dinner, he loosens up and has fun. He's great to travel with or to be around when he shows off his home or his collection of anitiques and paintings. We've spent some beautiful times together. On the other hand, we've also had some times when we were in strict business dealings that were not so pleasant. I'd seen that from the start, though; and I was always firm, always forceful. I knew I couldn't rely on him to put my welfare above his own, for which I couldn't blame him. It's always foolish in business to say, "Oh, he's my friend, he's going to take care of me." I'd been burned a few times in business before; I'd been taken advantage of in Munich, and I was determined not to let it happen again. Consequently I had to be as tough as Joe was when we did our dealing. A number of bodybuilders have not been as cautious and have found themselves backed into a corner because they thought, "Joe was really nice yesterday. He bought me a steak dinner. So he'll give me a fair shake when we sign the contract." But that's not so. Business and friendship are two different things for Joe, as they should be.

I think Joe is just naturally suspicious. He sometimes even feels his best friends are out to take advantage of him. Consequently, it's almost impossible to get him to trust you in business. It was always frustrating for me because he would seem to forget a lot of things he promised and I would be forced to remind him of them. We had seven years of ups and downs. But I'm proud of that fact that I remained with him and that, because of my tenacity, it was a good experience. There is nobody who's had a longer relationship with Joe Weider than I've had. And I don't believe anyone's come out better.

The reason it worked was honesty. That was my policy with Joe from the beginning—and my policy with anything, bodybuilding, business, anything. Instead of just talking behind his back, I said what I felt right to his face. Which he didn't always like, but which worked to solidify our relationship in the long run. If I didn't like something he did I told him point-blank. And he was the same with me.

Joe has played a big part in my life. He's partially responsible for my business mind and my success in business. I learned a lot from him, and I appreciate that. He helped make it possible for me to remain in America and work my way on to the top.

The first year people said I was really in shape was 1969. *Muscle Builder* magazine for May had my photograph on the cover. "Arnold Schwarzenegger—New Muscular Phenomenon." I trimmed down from 250 pounds to 230 pounds, which was a mind-blower for me because I was always pushing for gains, to be big. I couldn't maintain that mass any more; I was in heavy, heavy competition with the best bodybuilders in the world. This time I had to turn toward perfection. I had to reprogram my thinking: the best is not the biggest but the most perfectly developed. I had realized this painfully with my defeat by Frank Zane, and had started chiseling down. However, I knew that I had an advantage over most bodybuilders: when you have the size, the whole rough cut, you can sculpt it into a masterpiece—which was the major thrust of my work this whole year. I cut down and cut down and cut down; I chiseled and polished, rendering that animal mass I'd brought from Europe down to the work of art I wanted. I had jewel-like abdominals for the first time; it was the first time I knew there was such a thing as a low-carbohydrate diet. I'd never heard of special diets in Germany. There you ate and worked and grew.

One year in California had converted me to the cult that held it was the bodybuilder's paradise. The sunshine, the sea air and the moderate climate made it ideal for maintaining a body like mine. I loved Gold's Gym and the long, open stretches of beach, where I could run and then plunge into the sea for a swim.

Gold's Gym attracted the absolute best bodybuilders. It was almost an inspiration to work out there. A few weeks before any prestigious contest the noise level in the place would rise markedly. There would be less talk and more stone concentration. Cables would burn and sing through pulleys; steel plates would clank and ring; the weights lifted and dropped endlessly in the machines. It was like the background music for some ritual chant.

When I got to New York City that fall for the IFBB Mr. Universe contest I was cut and chiseled and tanned and could feel myself glowing. I reviewed the lineup. One guy wasn't there. This was Sergio Oliva, the Cuban bodybuilder, known as "the Myth," who had won the Mr. Olympia for two years in a row. He was considered the top man, the best in the business. But he was competing in the Mr. Olympia contest, which was being held that same night. All this cat-and-mouse stuff made me furious. I went to the officials and asked if there was still time for me to enter the Mr. Olympia competition. They agreed to let me in. I said to myself, Tonight I'm going to wipe him off too, because it's monkey business to keep going around in circles.

I won the IFBB Mr. Universe contest easily. Seven out of seven judges gave me first place. All during the judging I had the feeling it was all merely preparation for the Mr. Olympia contest. Now, as far as I was

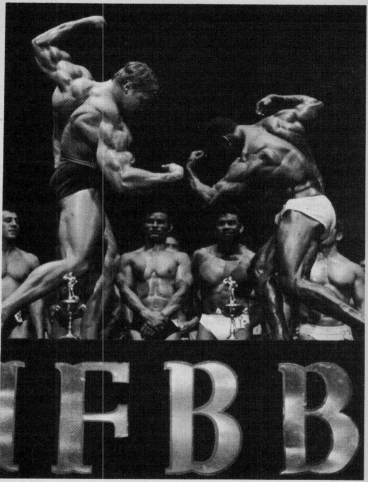

Pose-offs at my third Mr. Universe contest (IFBB), 1969

concerned, I had beat almost everybody in the world—except this black guy, Sergio Oliva.

I rushed to the Mr. Olympia contest. I entered the dressing room the way I'd been going in everyplace lately, like I was just taking over. Then, for the first time, I saw Sergio Oliva in person. I understood why they called him the Myth. It was as jarring, as if I'd walked into a wall. He destroyed me. He was so huge, he was so fantastic, there was no way I could even think of beating him. I admitted my defeat and felt some of my pump go away. I tried. But I'd been so taken back by my first sight of Sergio Oliva that I think I settled for second place before we walked out on the stage.

Interestingly enough, Sergio beat me only four to three, and that was a surprise. I thought he should have beat me seven to zero.

I never like to admit defeat, but I thought Sergio was better. There were no two ways about it. Though maybe he was not that much better. And that thought gave me energy to continue training, to go for another year. Again, I wasn't going to let up, and I made up my mind to return to the gym without a break. I fixed in my mind the image of Sergio. For a whole year, each time I felt lethargic, each time I felt myself weakening under the weight, I flashed on that image. I was going to destroy the Myth.

A week later was the Mr. Universe contest of the other federation (NABBA), in London. They were always a week apart. I flew to London because there were certain American bodybuilders who had gone to compete in this Mr. Universe. They wanted to get away from me and start competing in other contests— so they could win. I knew I was making my mark.

I showed up unexpectedly and I beat everybody there, winning my second Mr. Universe title in a single year. I had now won Mr. Universe four times. But there was still Sergio Oliva and the Mr. Olympia title. I had to beat Sergio. I went to Weider and said, "I'm

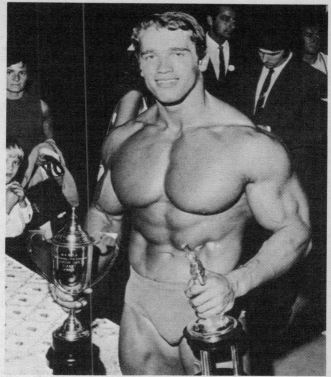

My fourth Mr. Universe victory (NABBA), 1969

pissed off, Joe. I want to stay another year, train as hard as possible, and beat Sergio."

Weider was pleased to have me remain in America. I talked him into bringing over Franco Columbu. It was important for me to be with Franco during a time when I wanted to adhere to a grueling workout schedule. Franco and I had become extremely close friends in Munich, and during my previous year of training in California without him I'd felt something was missing. Franco was largely into power training. I was training

mostly for definition and symmetry. The result of our
working together was the best possible training combination. Now Franco himself was hungry for winning.
Together, we trained harder than ever before, spend-
ing long, hard hours in the gym.

I did everything for refinement, for absolute perfection. I kept my diet strict. I used food supplements to
regulate the proper amounts of protein and vitamins
and minerals. I spent hours working out. I pushed myself past the limits of pain. I went to a dancer at UCLA
and started taking ballet lessons to further improve my
posing. This dancer showed me how to move my
hands gracefully, when a hand should be opened and
when it should be closed. We talked about what a fist
represents, what an open hand represents, how you
should move for the greatest impact, using your hands
as a signal. For instance, if you start a circular movement you should open your hand, and if you come
down in a sweeping movement you should close it in a
fist. All this helps give grace to your posing routine.
And grace is one thing people don't expect from a big
guy like me. That's why it's kind of shocking when I'm
onstage posing and I move and flow into this smooth,
super-graceful catlike routine. It definitely has a positive effect on the judges.

For some reason in 1970 the order of things was
reversed. The NABBA Mr. Universe contest was
scheduled in London a week *before* the IFBB Mr. Universe and Mr. Olympia contests. I went to London
first and had the shock of my life. One of my competitors was Reg Park, my idol. Over twenty years
after his debut in bodybuilding, he had trained a year
and staged a comeback.

I couldn't believe it. Here I was competing against
my idol, whose pictures I'd hung up all over my bedroom, whose words I'd lived and trained by. Thinking
about it left me with this weird, unreal sensation. I said
to myself, "There are two possibilities open to you:

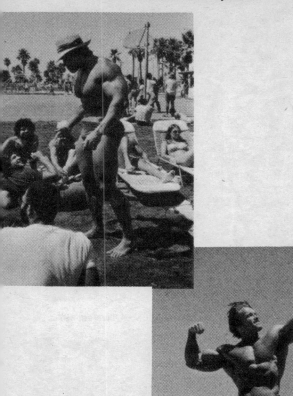

Fun at Venice Beach

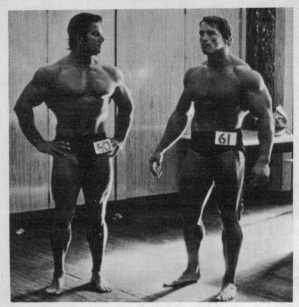

Competing with Reg Park for NABBA Mr. Universe, 1970

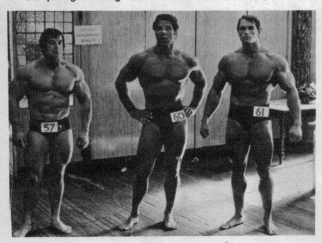

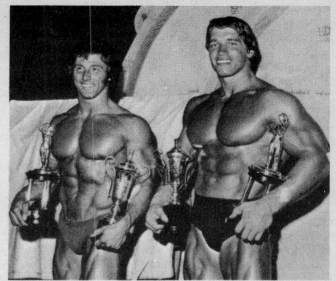

Posing with Frank Zane after winning my fifth Mr. Universe title

one is to beat Reg, and you most likely will, and destroy your idol; and the other is to leave London and not compete at all." I decided that leaving was stupid. It would be good for my ego and good for publicity to compete against Reg, to destroy my idol and win. We were both competitors, sportsmen, and there was a dignity in that. I didn't look at it as beating Reg Park but as being able to step up beside him, to finally share an equal place with him.

I entered the competition and I did beat him. He placed second, and Dave Draper third. It was one of the toughest Mr. Universes ever witnessed. It was the hardest year, period. Everybody went to London, Reg Park, Dave Draper, Boyer Coe and Dennis Tinnerino.

One day later the Mr. World contest was being held in Columbus, Ohio. All the eligible contestants flew immediately to New York. The contest officials picked us up in a private jet to insure our making it to Columbus on time. Another shock: Sergio Oliva was there. I hadn't expected him yet. I thought Mr. World would be an easy win and then I could go on to the Mr. Olympia contest two weeks later in New York and then face Sergio. At that point I wasn't sure I was ready for him, mentally. But I was feeling really strong after beating Reg Park and all the other previous Mr. Universe title holders, and I figured I was well on my way. My momentum was up. I had to do it. "Now's the time, Arnold," I told myself. "Screw you, Sergio. You can't bug me any more. This time I'm going to take over."

We started pumping up and getting ready. I kept watching Sergio, comparing our bodies in the mirrors. I was not wiped out, as I had been the year before. Sergio looked good. He had the kind of body that from the waist up seems as though it will never quit getting bigger. But I was cut, just really perfect. Everything was really in—separation, definition, everything—and I felt confident. I went onstage with the host and was met with tremendous applause. I didn't know where it was coming from. It was a total surprise. Ohio? Nobody thinks of Ohio as a fan's state. But the applause continued and any apprehension I had fled.

I felt the pressure so deeply the prejudging and the show seemed to blend in my mind. It became all one fantastic push forward. I felt taller, bigger, more muscular, more graceful. I got high from the force of the pump. I felt as though I stepped out of my body to watch. I never felt the flame of competition more strongly. I was glad for the year of savage workouts Franco and I had put in; otherwise I could not have withstood the intensity I created during the final pose-off. The audience itself seemed miles away. I limited my scope to the microcosm of the stage—Arnold and Sergio.

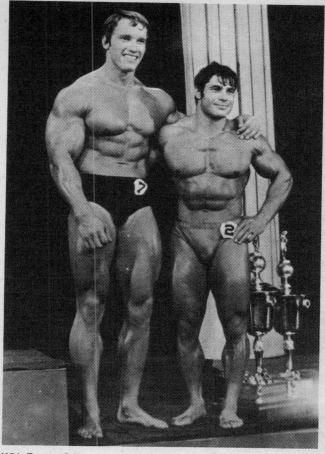

With Franco Columbu at the 1970 Mr. World contest, Columbus, Ohio

The announcer cleared his throat and rustled a pile of papers. "In third place," he said, "Dave Draper."

The audience grew silent. "Second place," the announcer said, pausing . . ."Sergio Oliva." Beside me, I heard Sergio say, "Oh, shit!"

There it was, then, that cry again: "Arnold! Arnold!" I had won. In a single second, I had taken the final step. I had conquered every great bodybuilder in the world.

I hated Sergio's attitude. It's tough to lose, but that's no reason to be a poor loser. I watched him, thinking, "Last year you beat me, Sergio. I got you tonight and I'll get you again in two weeks." That gave me even more momentum to go to New York.

This contest, the Mr. Olympia, was billed as the bodybuilding battle of the century. I had won Mr. World in Ohio, but that had been so close that two weeks in the gym could change the outcome. In New York the camps were split. It was a competition solely between Sergio and me.

I was never quite so aware of what fanatics there are in the bodybuilding audience as I was then. They seemed to cling to me. I couldn't go anyplace without people clustering around to touch me. The closer it got to contest time, the more frantic they became. It was a madness. First it was autographs; then clothing. The requests got more bizarre. Word reached me that someone was offering a hundred dollars for a lock of my hair, five hundred for my posing trunks.

In the dressing room, Sergio was already pumping up. I didn't take my eyes off him. But I didn't even make a move to change. I just watched him. I followed each move he made with my eyes. He'd pause and look around at me, to see if I'd started to strip down. I knew it was getting to him. Finally, with two minutes to go, I slipped into my trunks and oiled up.

Police were having to keep the fans from the stage. They had gone berserk. Some were screaming, "Sergio!" But "Arnold!" cut through and put them down.

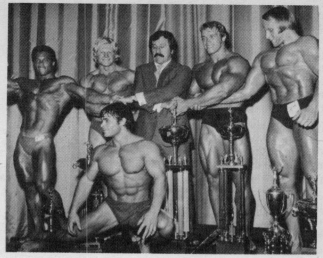

Winning Mr. Olympia, 1970—from left: Rick Wayne, Dave Draper, Joe Weider, myself, Mike Katz, and Franco Columbu in front

All the sheer madness of a stampede came out in those fans. They were holding up photographs, waving banners, trying to get to the stage only to be pushed back and threatened by ushers and cops.

The moment the announcer gave me the title and the girl handed me the trophy and I clutched the cold silver bowl against my stomach I knew I had gone as far as I could in bodybuilding as a competitor. From then on I would only be defending my title, and that put things in a whole different light. I had cleaned house. That was it. It's what I call the golden triangle. I went boom, boom, boom in three cities in two weeks. I beat everybody, every formidable contender who ever existed in bodybuilding. I was King Kong. The Mr. Olympia contest is the Super Bowl of bodybuilding. I had reached the point where I wanted to be. I no longer needed the ego satisfaction of winning, winning, winning. But I was excited too. This was what I was actually looking forward to more than anything anyway. Because I'd begun to look at bodybuilding as a kind of vehicle. It feels good being the best-built man in the world, of course, but the question always comes up: Okay, how can you use that to make money? I had been increasingly more involved in business since the year I bought the gym. I no longer had to prove I was the greatest bodybuilder of all time. Now I had to reach out to the general public, to people who knew nothing about bodybuilding, and educate them to the benefits of weight training.

I'd always loved the excitement of winning, but I loved it especially when there was a contest. It seemed to me that I had made my mark in bodybuilding. I knew there were other contests, other worlds to conquer. I was already into business, and I was working and studying to get into acting. My acting classes opened up an entire new space for me: myself. One thing I learned was to look back and analyze who I was and what I'd done.

Working in the same way I had to build my body, I wanted to create an empire. Because of my business education and the practical aspects of business I learned from Joe Weider, I felt I was equipped to go ahead with my own enterprises. I established a series of mail-order training courses which enabled me to help educate thousands of bodybuilders all over the world. I sold photo albums, tee shirts, posing trunks, personalized programs. I worked out seminars all over the world—Japan, Australia, South Africa, Holland, Belgium, Germany, Austria, Italy, France, Finland, Spain, Canada, Mexico and the United States. I began promoting bodybuilding competitions in America. In order to keep up my name and make it grow, I continued to defend my titles. Eventually, I wanted every single person who touched a weight to equate the feeling of the barbell with my name. The moment he got a hold of it I wanted him to think, "Arnold."

I think the most important things I developed through bodybuilding were my personality, confidence and character. When you have a well-developed body and you're confident, you see people bending your way, wanting to be on your side, wanting to do things for you. When I was young I suffered from the same insecurity every kid has. But as I transformed myself into something strong and unique, discovering I could do one thing well, confidence came to me naturally. And that gave me a great deal of security.

I believe you overcome a lot of frustrations in the gymnasium, things you're not even aware of. I found that the more I worked out, the less violent I became. It trimmed away tensions and taught me how to relax: When I put in a good workout I felt a sense of accomplishment. I felt like a newborn person. I had the strength to go on and conquer in other areas and feel confident about doing it. It left me in kind of a low-key frame of mind, not always desperate or anxious. Every day, I see people running around, all excited, wanting to do things, feeling pent up and unable to find any release. I'd probably be that way if I didn't work off my frustrations in the gym. I've come to realize that almost anything difficult, any challenge, takes time, patience and hard work, like building up for a 300-pound bench press. Learning that gave me plenty of positive energy to use later on.

I taught myself discipline, the strictest kind of discipline. How to be totally in control of my body, how to control each individual muscle. I could apply that discipline to everyday life. I used it in acting, in going to school. Whenever I didn't want to study I would just think back and remember what it took to be Mr. Universe—the sacrifice, the hard work—and I would plunge myself into studying.

Bodybuilding changed me entirely. I think I would be a different person now if I'd never trained, if I'd just worked somewhere. It gave me confidence and pride and an unlimited positive attitude. I can apply my success to everything. One thing is that people listen much more to bigger guys; the bigger you are and the more impressive you look physically, the more people listen and the better you can sell yourself or anything else. In business school I saw a study of how many big companies in America hire salesmen above a certain height and weight. Because it has been proved that big people are more impressive salespeople. They're more convincing. It's true. I found it out myself, that I can persuade people easier than a small person can.

I've had no problem making it work. I just looked back at how I did it in bodybuilding and then applied it to other things. With acting, now, I am determined to work as hard on removing my accent as I was on improving my poor calves. The same with business. I'm so determined to make millions of dollars that I cannot fail. In my mind I've already made the millions; now it's just a matter of going through the motions.

Not the least reward of a fit body is continuous good health. As a very small child I was constantly sick. Even later on I spent a part of every year in bed with a heavy cold. Since I began bodybuiding, in the last fourteen years, I have only been sick two or three times, and then it was only a minor cold. I have developed a perfect communication between my body and my mind; I have total control over my body. My body responds better; I fight off things easier. My body has become like a clock, a special clock that is tuned so well it only goes wrong one second in five years. That's how I feel about my body. It is so perfect that everything works. And I very rarely see other bodybuilders getting sick. There are fewer heart attacks among bodybuilders because blood is being pumped through the veins so hard it keeps the veins open; and when you pump up the muscles it pumps

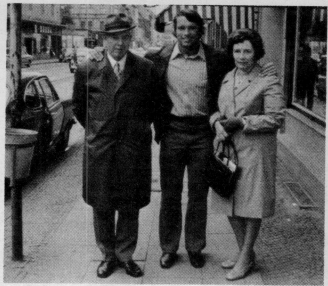

With my parents in Munich

blood through them and trains the heart every time you train. My own circulation is fantastic.

During all the years I was into heavy competition I avoided any kind of binding relationship, although I saw a lot of women. Then in 1969 I met a girl who changed my thinking. Her name was Barbara; she was a waitress in Zuckie's in Santa Monica, working there during the summer to help pay for schooling at San Diego State. I asked her out and was impressed immediately by something I felt about her, something that was different from most of the girls I had been dating. I could describe it as an inner warmth, the wholesomeness one associates with a hometown girl. Our dating was different, too, from any I'd ever done. She took me to meet her parents. This also impressed me. There was a healthy atmosphere in their home. They seemed to have communication. They felt love and respect for each other and expressed it.

Barbara liked me as a human being, not as a bodybuilder, as Mr. Universe. In fact, she knew nothing about the sport and didn't find out that I had any titles until weeks after we met. I was just Arnold, we were going out, and she was helping me with my English. She genuinely cared about me. I felt love coming from her.

We dated until the end of August, when she went back to San Diego and I left for Europe. While I was gone, the one person I thought about was Barbara. I talked about her and even wrote to her, which was unheard of for me. My friends started kidding me: "Arnold's in love." I was surprised that other people could see that in me.

I returned to America in October, but I remained in New York City until mid-December. I caught myself talking about Barbara, wanting her. I called her from New York and made plans to meet her as soon as I got back to California.

All the way back on the plane I had these mixed emotions—what was wrong with me? Why did I continue to talk of this girl? All I knew was that with her I had allowed something to happen that I had guarded against for years. There was something else there besides a diversion, a release. I actually wanted to be with her.

It was an unusual experience for me. I began to explore my feelings, to see why this was happening. I would pull away and watch myself. I had taught myself always to pull back and look at whatever I was doing and make a judgment about it. I always tried to be honest. It baffled me now to see that I was enjoying something more than a physical relationship with someone. I liked it. And I was happy. I had found someone who loved me, who really cared for me.

Two years later, when she had finished school and could come to Santa Monica permanently, we decided to move in together. It was her suggestion, but I was instantly agreeable. Again I saw new changes in myself. I was enjoying the experience of putting together an apartment—a place for living, not just some pad where I could sleep, hang out.

Gradually a conflict grew up in our relationship. Basically it came down to this: she was a well-balanced woman who wanted an ordinary, solid life, and I was not a well-balanced man and hated the very idea of ordinary life. She had thought I would settle down, that I would reach the top in my field and level off. But that's a concept that has no place in my thinking. For me, life is continuously being hungry. The meaning of life is not simply to exist, to survive, but to move ahead, to go up, to achieve, to conquer. When she saw me moving away from bodybuilding into another challenging field, acting, I think she realized we could not go on together. When I went to Alabama to begin the filming of *Stay Hungry,* she moved to her own apartment.

That was a tough time for me. I was torn between two things. I felt that a part of me had been ripped right out of my body. I had lost something good, something that had helped hold me together. Barbara had taught me how to appreciate a woman. Emotionally, I wanted to stay with her. Intellectually, I knew it would never work. I wanted to grow, to go on; the life she wanted wouldn't permit that. I had learned how a relationship can be beautiful, how it can add to the meaning of your life and feed your soul.

I've retired from bodybuilding but I haven't quit. I have only stopped competing. I would describe myself as sort of the leader of the bodybuilders. Many times I feel like I'm their mother. They come to me with all their problems. They write me about their problems.

Every year before competitions they ask me where they should compete and at what body weight, what posing trunks to wear, what oil to use, and how to pose. They want advice about contract negotiations and the stories they want to write for muscle magazines.

I become very emotionally attached to them every summer, during the time of training, when I work out with them. Whoever you are training with, the two of you become like one unit—it's like being married for three months—and you do almost everything together: you go out to eat together, you train together, you lie in the sun together, you spend free time together talking, trying to inspire each other. You become attached to each other.

I'm always the leader, because I'm the more outgoing personality, I'm a domineering person. And I'm also the most experienced bodybuilder, the one who has had the most success. I've traveled all over the world, I've done hundreds and hundreds of exhibitions. I've only lost three competitions—and each time it was second place. So they look up to me.

For many of them I'm the hero, and that's why I've become a caretaker. Especially now that I am out of competition and into promoting competitions. It's a whole different ballgame, because I think bodybuilders see me as a person who loves bodybuilding and is really trying to help it as a sport. I am trying to do this by running the top shows, the Mr. Olympia and Mr. Universe competitions. I want to bring more money into bodybuilding and see that the competitors get a greater share of it.

Whatever else I do, I want to always be a kind of ambassador, a preacher for bodybuilding.

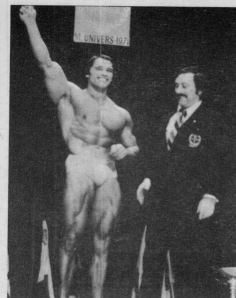

Mr. Olympia, 1971; with Joe Weider

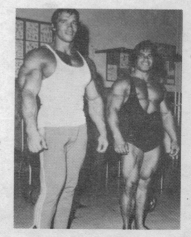

With Ed Corney

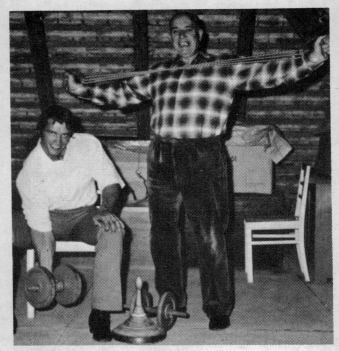

Training with Father

Mr. Olympia, 1973; with Joe Weider

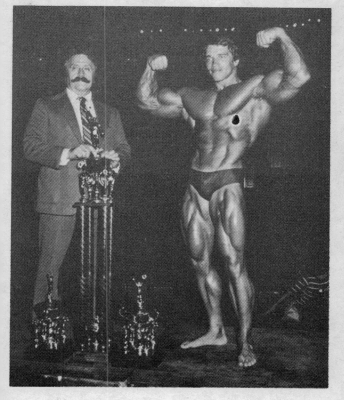

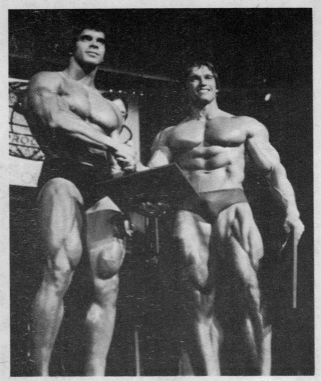

Mr. Olympia, after beating Lou Ferrigno; 1974

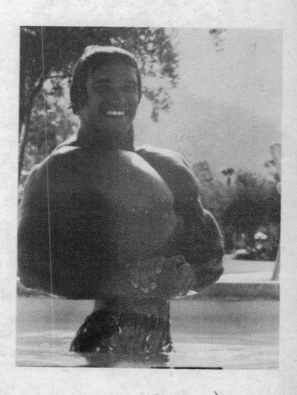

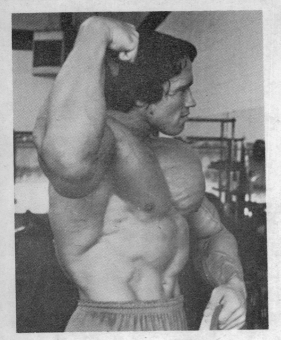

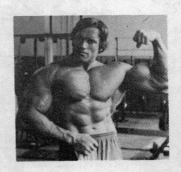

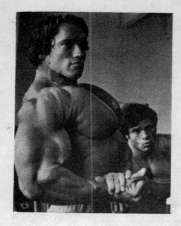

Practicing posing

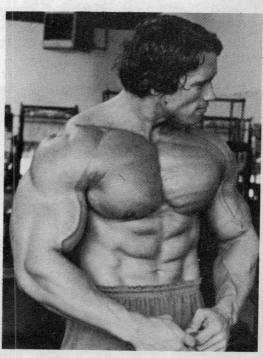

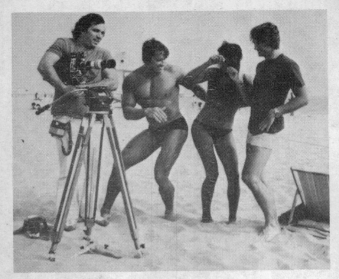

Fooling around during the filming of *Pumping Iron*

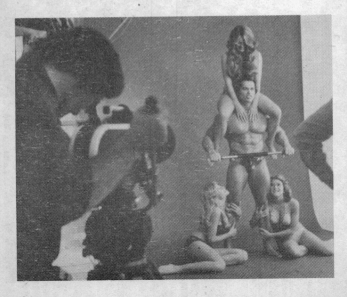

Courtesy of United Artists

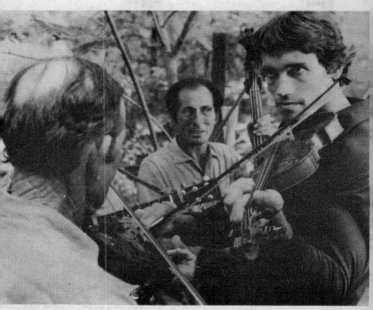

Learning to play the violin during shooting of *Stay Hungry*

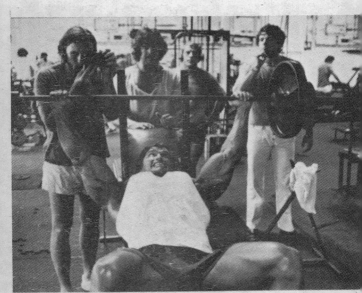

Working out in top form, 1973

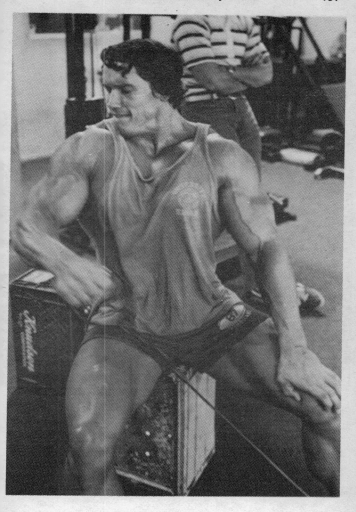

Prejudging poses for Mr. Olympia, 1974

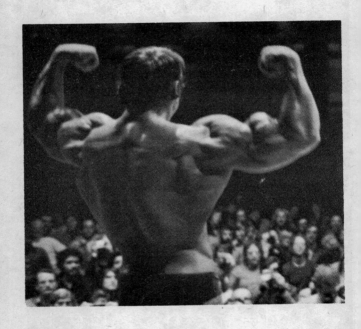

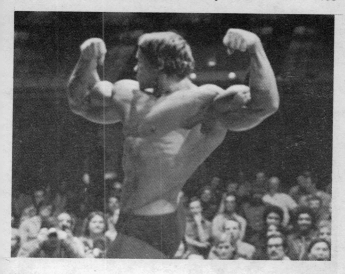

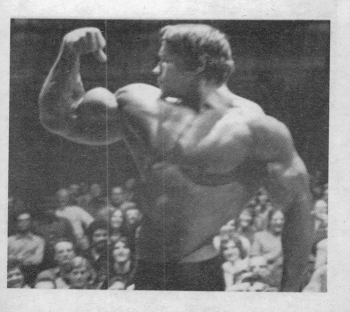

Posing on a mountain in California called Muscle Rock, 1974. All the top bodybuilders of the past thirty years have been photographed on this spot.

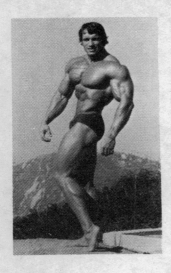

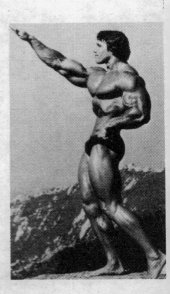

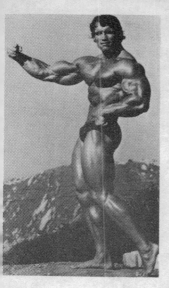

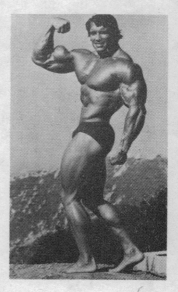

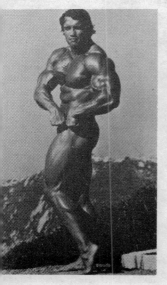

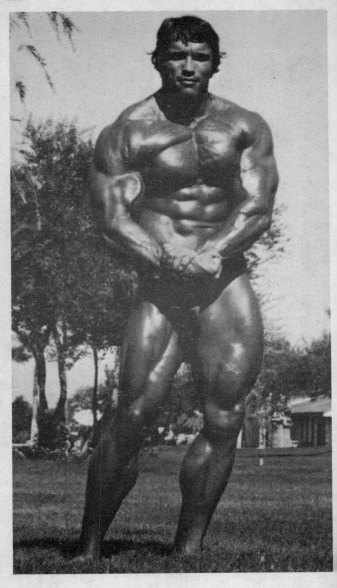

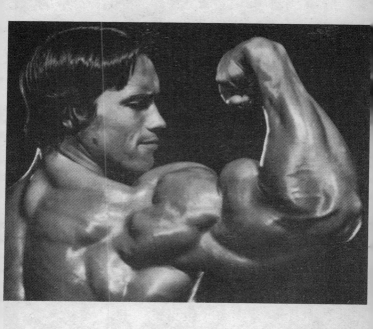

Palm Springs, 1974

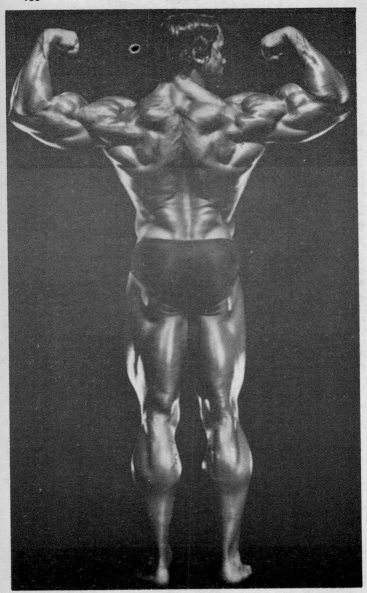

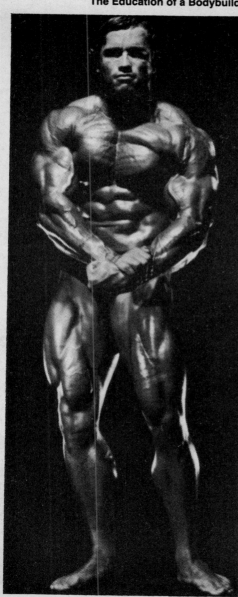

Studio posing,
1974

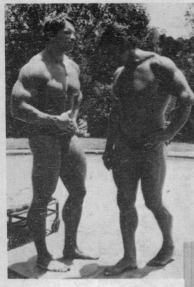

Oiling up

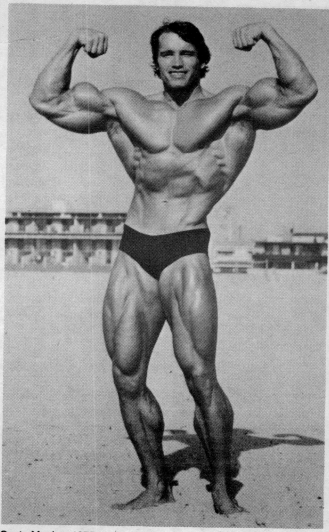

Santa Monica, 1975

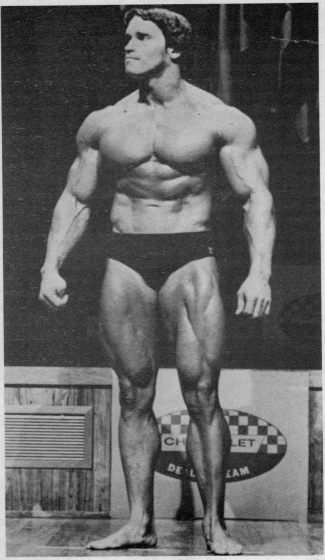

Prejudging for Mr. Olympia, South Africa, 1975

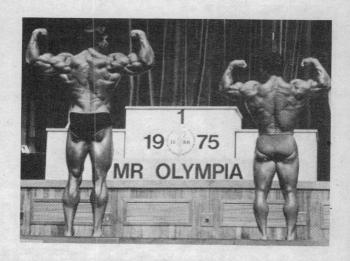

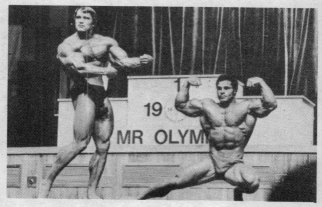

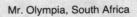

Mr. Olympia, South Africa

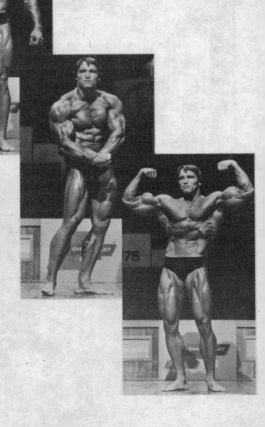

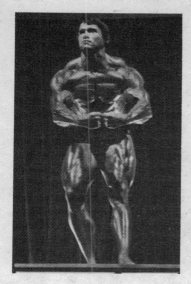

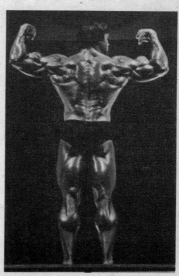

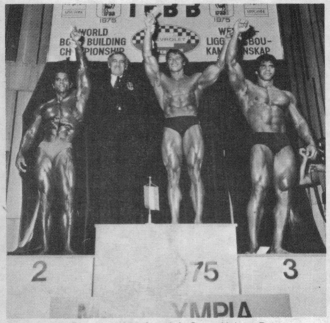

Victory—Mr. Olympia, 1975; from left: Serge Nubret, Ben Weider (President of IFBB), myself, Lou Ferrigno

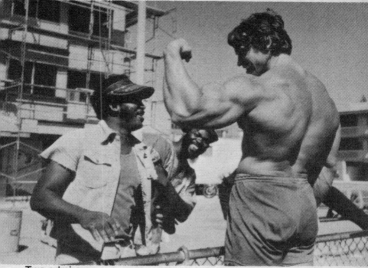

Two admirers

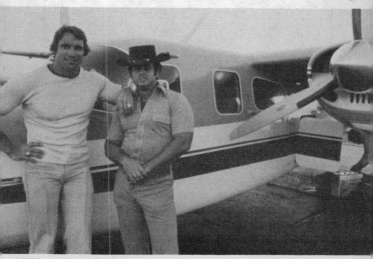

With my friend Bill Drake, who helped me very much when I first came to America

The pictures on the following pages are my favorite photos of my competitive posing routine

Top Form Measurements

Arms	22 inches
Chest	57 inches
Waist	34 inches
Thighs	28½ inches
Calves	20 inches
Weight	235 pounds
Height	6 feet 2 inches

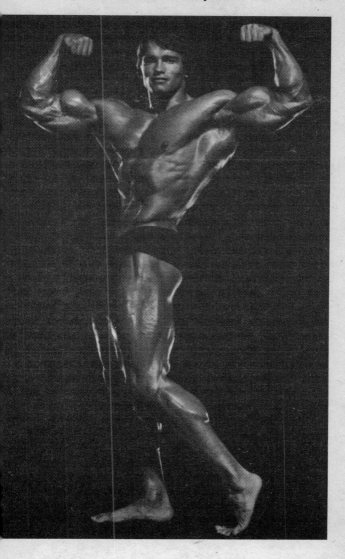

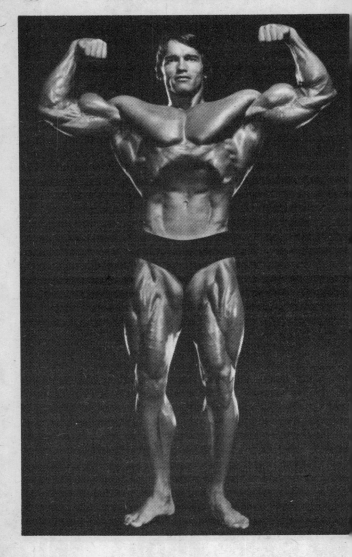

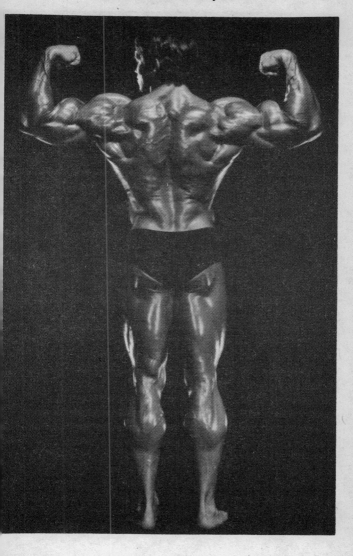

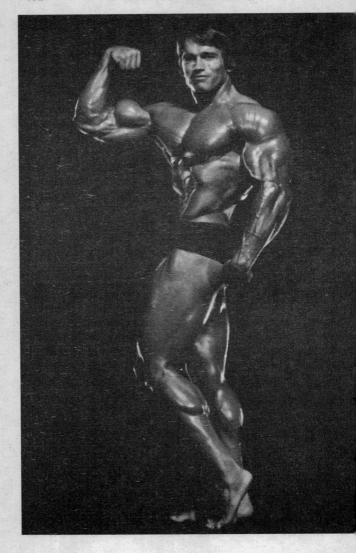

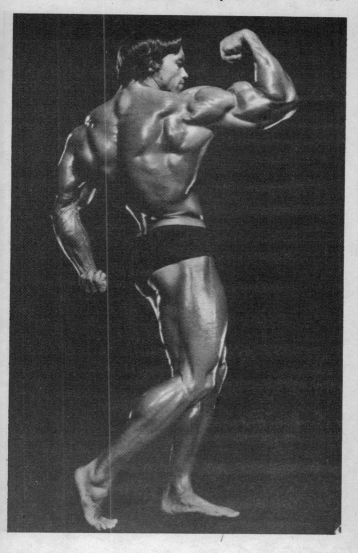

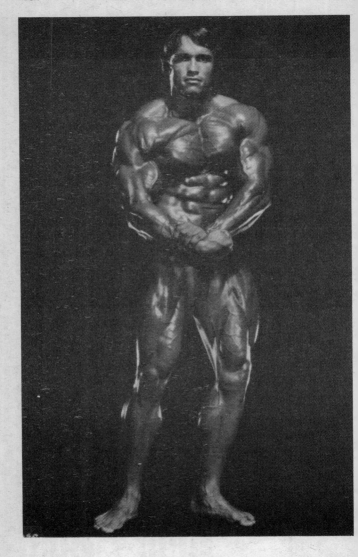

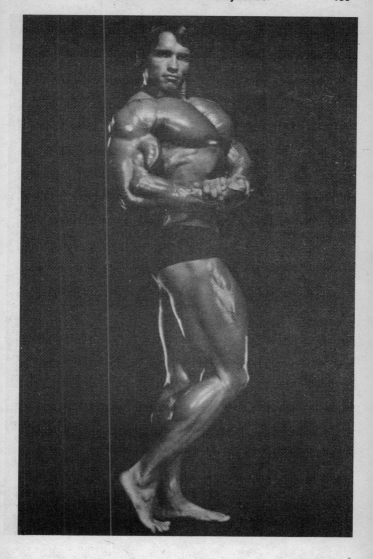

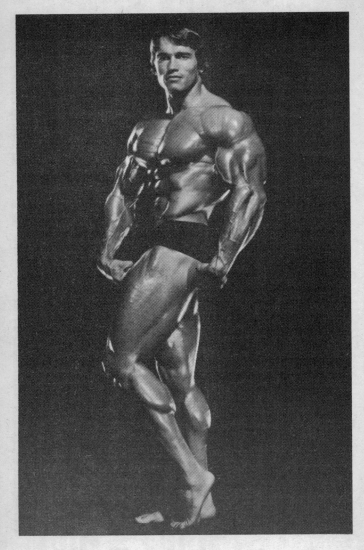

PART TWO
Muscles

Chapter One
Introduction

There is nothing as good as bodybuilding to get your body tuned up and totally in shape. It doesn't matter whether you want speed or brute strength, whether you want to run or develop endurance power. The only activity that can build the entire body evenly and uniformly is progressive weight resistance training.

Twenty years ago there was a widespread negative attitude toward bodybuilding. A lot of coaches and other people connected with the various sports claimed it was not the right kind of training for athletes, that it was just to look big and massive and muscular. They equated size and muscularity with awkwardness. All bodybuilders were said to be musclebound. It has now been proved that bodybuilding and weight resistance training are valuable for every purpose. Today we find weight rooms in high schools and universities. These are used by all kinds of athletes from runners to baseball players. In fact, in the last ten years, professional football teams all across the United States have made incredible advances through pre-season programs in weight training. Recently, I asked Brian Oldfield what advantages weight lifting had given him, and he said his ability to put the shot farther and with more accuracy was directly connected to the increase in pounds of weight he lifted while training in the gym. Karl Schranz, a skier with a body weight of only 160 pounds, went on television and demonstrated the 400-pound squats he did for his legs. O. J. Simpson was able to win the Superstar games with the extra points he won from weight lifting. It works for the guy who builds his body to be Mr. Universe, for someone who simply wants to trim down his stomach and broaden his shoulders a little bit, or for someone who needs to improve his circulation. Weight training is being used more and more for physical therapy following orthopedic operations. Its benefits go far beyond physical fitness. Bobby Fischer lifted weights to help him feel more confident before the world championships in chess.

Weight resistance training develops every muscle in your body. Which is not something you can say for any other sport. Take tennis, for example. After you've played for some time, your legs will develop; but nothing significant happens to your shoulders, back, chest, or abdominal muscles. I discovered a similar thing when I was skiing. I built up incredible endurance in my legs, but my arms and upper body stayed weak. In other words, in almost every sport there are some muscles, some areas of the body, that are neglected. But I can promise you one thing about progressive resistance weight training: if you are doing your workouts properly, after a short time you will notice that you not only feel and look better, but that your tennis, golf, skiing, swimming or whatever will be greatly improved. You'll have better stamina, agility, coordination and resilience.

The General Nature of Exercise

One very good reason to train is that the body doesn't get enough physical activity to keep it tuned and responsive. A hundred years ago we had to do everything with our bodies. We had to walk to a farm to get milk, we worked to get lumber and stones for building a house. We had to work with our hands, we had to run, we had to crawl under things, we had to swim. The efforts of everyday living kept the body in shape. But now, because almost everything is done with machines, people have become lazy. I'm as guilty as anyone: I drive my car a block to the supermarket to buy food.

If we don't have any exercise to stimulate the muscles, they deteriorate. That's why today there are lots of needless injuries. People pick up something heavy and pull the muscles in their backs. Housewives make a bed and dislocate a shoulder. Guys try to change a tire and rip a bicep. Why? Because the body isn't prepared. This alone is a very good reason to do some kind of bodybuilding.

In the human body there are over 600 muscles, which are made up of approximately 100 billion muscle fibers; we are not even aware of many of these muscles, muscles that make the fingers close and give you a strong grip, muscles that open the eyelid, muscles that work so automatically you've never even felt them before. In fact, the human body is more than half muscle. Muscles are used in every movement we make. They propel food along the digestive tract, suck air into the lungs, tighten blood vessels to raise blood pressure when needed to meet an emergency. The thing that first turned me on to bodybuilding was realizing that through weight resistance exercises I could stimulate each muscle in the body. I could be in control of it and not merely a victim of its weaknesses.

Most people are aware only of muscles that they use in everyday work. But when you do unusual movements or use your body in unusual ways, you feel muscles you never knew existed. I've seen people who have climbed a mountain for the first time—ten miles of hiking and climbing—and the next day they came down and said, "Wow, my calves hurt . . . my lower back is stiff." It was the first time they'd felt their calves or lower back in their whole lives. They'd never even thought of themselves as having muscles in those places.

I remember once my mother was lifting up the heavy mattresses to make a bed and she pulled her bicep. It was the first time she was conscious of having a bicep. And at the same time she was horrified that I was into weight training, that I was eager to stay in shape, to avoid such injuries.

Most people prefer to let their muscles remain anonymous. They take it for granted that the body just moves. Then they are baffled when something goes wrong. One of the benefits of bodybuilding is that it makes you aware of all your muscles. You start getting sore in certain parts of the body when you train. You realize what an incredibly complex machine the body is. For that reason, it's very important when you're doing your first workouts, laying the foundation for future training, that you are really sensitive and tuned in to the soreness. Remember the soreness and connect it in your mind with the exercise you were doing. This will help you later on to know that when you train certain areas you should concentrate on a specific kind of exercise and do it in a specific way. From the very start you should look on soreness as positive, as a sign of building, of growth.

Mind and Body

You must consider that in the beginning you are training the mind as well as the body. The mind, after all, makes you want to train; it turns on the body. Because the mind motivates you to train the body, you have to train the mind first. If the mind doesn't want to lift weights, the body won't lift them.

The mind is incredible. Once you've gained mastery over it, channeling its powers *positively* for your purposes, you can do anything. I mean anything. The secret is to make your mind work for you—not against you. This means constantly being positive, constantly setting up challenges you can meet—either today, next week, or next month. "I can't . . ." should be permanently stricken from your vocabulary, especially the vocabulary of your thoughts. You must see yourself always growing and improving.

You should strive to improve your body a little bit at a time. Don't push the mind too much either; let the mind stay hungry for more, tease the mind a little bit. This is why I suggest you start small, with a fairly easy program. Let the body say to the mind, "I feel good, this isn't too hard. I'm ready for more!" Give it more, give it a little bit more. Then, slowly, as the mind is ready for it, you can increase the amount of weight you use and the number of repetitions you do of an exercise.

A Reason

You should know why you are going to start training. This is one of the most important steps in initiating a successful bodybuilding program. You should not go to the gym because somebody says, "Hey, you're a slob. You ought to do some weight training and get in shape." That isn't a good reason, because you would be trying to satisfy someone else's wishes, not your own. You should have a very good reason why *you* want to get into weight resistance training. The best thing to do is to sit down and say to yourself, "What do I want to get out of it? What is my goal?"

Be honest. Honesty is the key to how much you can improve. Your reason could be that you want to be a bodybuilder, a competitive bodybuilder. That will certainly get you started training. But even if you only want to lose a few inches around the waist, you should be very explicit and spell it out for yourself. "The reason I want to do this weight training is that I want to lose this waist. I look in the mirror, it looks horrible." Or, "I'm a doctor and when my patients look at me I know they're thinking, 'What kind of example is he setting?' " Whatever your reason is, write it down and put it where you'll see it in the months to come.

Next you have to decide what you want to look like. Again, be explicit. My own image was Reg Park. I built it so clearly in my mind I could actually see myself standing in Reg Park's body. This second step, forming an image in the mind, creates what I call the want power. You have an image of what you want to look like, which in turn creates the willpower to go into the gym and work out. Now you have a goal. Without it you'd be like a ship without a destination. You must know why you are training in order to give it your best and be productive.

I conduct seminars all over the world, and the first thing I hear is: "Am I going to find out in this seminar how to do a curl?" "Will I find out how to do a bench press?" I say to them, "Wait a minute, the first hour will be just on what our goals are. Why we train. What makes us not go dancing in the evenings but go to the gymnasium instead and spend two hours doing workouts." A lot of people are confused about my reasoning; they think the exercises in the gym are the most important thing. But I maintain the most important thing is to be straight in your mind, to be honest with yourself. The exercises are the easy part.

Analyze Yourself—Be Realistic

Before you start working out it's very important to look at yourself and categorize yourself in terms of which of the three body types you are—ectomorph, endomorph, or mesomorph. Remember these are not rigid definitions. Most people are a combination of characteristics from more than one type. But the dominant characteristics are what you should be looking for in your assessment.

The Ectomorph: A thin person with a light bone

structure and long tenuous muscles. The ectomorph has a tough time gaining weight and building strength.

The Endomorph: A stocky person with thick bones and a general tendency to be round and stout. The endomorph will gain fast and be able to handle heavy training. His body is more likely to remain blocky and muscular without showing great cuts or definition.

The Mesomorph: Anatomically, the ideal body for weight resistance training. The mesomorph has a large frame and the capacity for becoming muscular fast.

You can improve your body. All that you should look for in training with weights is that you should achieve 100% of your potential. That potential varies greatly among three body types and individuals within each type.

If you are a skinny guy, an ectomorph, you are not really lost, though your kind of muscles are the most difficult to build. You may need to change your metabolism and perhaps correct a problem with your thyroid gland so you can start gaining weight—so, in a way, you're on the safe side.

If you're an endomorph, one of those round people who really don't have muscle tone to begin with, you should realize that your type of body will probably not go all the way to Mr. Universe. You won't have it as hard as the ectomorph, but you'll need to put more mental energy into it than the muscular type, the mesomorph. If you are a mesomorph, the athletic, muscular type, you are the one who might—if you have the right mental attitude—achieve a Mr. Universe physique.

Remember, these are generalizations. The power of the mind is astonishing. There may be an endomorph reading this page who adamantly disagrees with me. He has it in his head that he's going to become Mr. Universe and nothing Arnold can say will dissuade him. More power to him. If he believes it long enough and hard enough and matches his conviction with hard, relentless work, he might just make it.

What You Can Achieve with a Program of Regular Exercise

If you exercise faithfully, with a strict adherence to form, you should notice an increase in strength and coordination within a very short time. Your joint mobility and flexibility will be better. You'll expend less energy in performing both physical and mental tasks. You'll have better posture. Your ability to relax and voluntarily reduce stress and tension will be heightened. Your heart should become stronger and your circulation improve. You'll have greater immunity from illness. You'll be better protected from injuries, and be able to heal more rapidly when one does occur.

Get a Physician's Checkup Prior to Beginning a Training Program

There is no age limit on improving your body and no body that cannot be improved by regular exercise. However, before anyone over the age of twenty-five engages in any form of strenuous exercise—including jogging, tennis, handball, etc.—a medical checkup is advisable. In all probability the doctor will give you a go-ahead. If you have some health problem, he can take proper measures to correct it, and he may have some useful suggestions or cautionary advice to help you modify the exercise program to make it more suitable and beneficial for you.

I think a physical exam is important. Not only will you find out whether or not your heart is sound, but you'll also be checked for other conditions you might have: low metabolism rate, thyroid problems, vitamin deficiency. These are things that affect how you lose or gain weight. They could put you off balance and make your body fail to respond favorably although you are training hard, eating right and getting sufficient sleep.

If you are physically active now and in reasonably good health, you can start on the exercises with little or no break-in period. If you are in poor physical condition and/or have been inactive for some time, then you should gradually build up to the full program.

Eating for Muscles

Every person who takes up bodybuilding should have a basic understanding of nutrition. The very words *body building* imply that we are undertaking something constructive. An exercise program is not enough. Exercise merely tones and develops existing muscles. In order to build muscles we must have the nutrients that promote growth. In this section I shall provide only a basic outline of what is involved in good eating. This should serve the needs of most people. If you have a special problem, you should consult a physician and study books on diet and nutrition.

There are three primary nutritional elements—proteins, carbohydrates and fats. They are all necessary to the well-balanced diet. I would suggest that in planning your diet you obtain a small calorie counter from your supermarket or drugstore. Be certain it gives a complete breakdown of the various foods—how many grams of protein, carbohydrates and fats are in each portion. Use it to help regulate your intake of body-building fuel.

Protein is the most important element to the bodybuilder. Protein is for growth, maintenance and repair of muscle tissue. The amount of protein needed by the average person is 1 gram for each 2 pounds of body weight. The bodybuilder needs more—approximately 1 gram of protein to each pound of body weight. Someone on a super-gain program will require even more protein—at least 1½ grams of protein for every pound of body weight.

The highest-quality proteins come from animal

sources—eggs, fish, poultry, meat and dairy products. Much lower in value (because they are not as readily assimilated) are proteins of plant origin—beans, rice, corn, peas and nuts. To make these more readily available for use in the body they should be taken with animal proteins. Generally speaking, the bodybuilder will experience the fastest growth by choosing proteins from animal sources.

Carbohydrates raise the blood sugar level and supply the muscles with energy. You need a certain amount of carbohydrates to fuel your system so it can utilize its available protein to the greatest advantage.

Fats too are essential to a good diet. Not only do they heat your body and lubricate your body parts, they also provide a necessary base for carrying vitamins A, D and E.

Aside from protein, carbohydrates and fats, you should have adequate vitamins and minerals. It is preferable to get your vitamins and minerals from the foods you eat. However, in accelerated training situations it is advisable to reinforce your regular diet with supplements. The following are the vitamins your body needs to maintain itself properly:

Vitamin A—important to good vision, skin texture, and maintaining the delicate linings of the nose and throat. Sources: eggs, liver, milk, carrots, spinach.

Vitamin B complex (twelve B vitamins, including niacin, riboflavin and thiamine)—essential to a good balance of the nervous system and the normal functioning of the digestive system. Sources: eggs, whole grains, poultry, green vegetables, fish, fruit, milk, brewer's yeast.

Vitamin C—promotes healing; builds up resistance to infection; aids in the production of connective tissues; generally strengthens the skeletal and vascular systems. Sources: citrus fruits, tomatoes, green vegetables.

Vitamin D—essential for strong teeth and bones.

Sources: milk, fish, egg yolks, chicken livers and, especially, direct sunlight.

Vitamin E—contributes to the functioning of the circulatory, respiratory and reproductive systems. Sources: wheat germ, vegetable oils, eggs and leafy green vegetables.

In addition to vitamins, and in many cases to make certain vitamins available to the body, you require adequate amounts of the following minerals: calcium, magnesium, phosphorus, iron, iodine, potassium, sodium, copper, zinc, manganese.

There are four basic food groups. You should be aware of these groups and see that you include something from each one in your daily diet.

1. Milk and dairy products—cheese, cottage cheese, yoghurt and buttermilk.
2. Fish, poultry, meat and eggs.
3. Fruits and vegetables (preferably fresh).
4. Breads, cereals, fats.

Obviously, you will concentrate on the first two groups, since they contain the high-protein foods. But do not neglect carbohydrates and fats. To maintain the stamina to train, you need fuel and energy foods.

One thing every bodybuilder (or individual concerned with the ultimate welfare of his body) ought to do is to cut super-refined foods and food products from his diet. Do yourself a favor: start eating foods that will give you quality and vitality. Replace all refined sugar with honey. Avoid cakes, pies, candies, french fries and packaged snacks. Satisfy your sweet tooth with fresh fruit.

Those readers who wish to lose weight can do so easily just by cutting out sweets, as I have suggested, balancing meals for more protein, and staying with the exercise program. However, if you really want to put on muscle I am including my super weight-gaining diet.

The secret of rapid weight gain is a high-protein, high-calorie diet. Your body can effectively utilize only so much protein at a time: 30 to 50 grams seems to be the maximum amount. Eating six small meals a day (instead of three large ones) is the ideal way to pace your protein intake. Smaller amounts of food are handled more easily by the digestive system, and there is no danger of over-stretching the stomach. The following diet is based on the frequent-small-meal principle and supplies just over 5,000 calories and 300 grams of protein.

BREAKFAST: 7:30 A.M.
    3 eggs; ¼- to ½-pound beef patty; 2 pieces buttered toast; 2 glasses milk

MIDMORNING SNACK: 10:00 A.M.
    half sandwich, meat; 1 hard-boiled egg; 1 glass milk

LUNCH: 12:30 P.M.
    1 meat sandwich; 1 cheese sandwich; 2 glasses milk; fruit

MIDAFTERNOON SNACK: 3:00 P.M.
    1 hard-boiled egg; 3 slices cheese; 2 glasses milk

SUPPER: 6:00 P.M.
    ½ to ¾ pound ground beef; baked potato with butter; salad; vegetable (corn, beans, peas, etc.); 2 glasses milk

BEDTIME SNACK: 9:00 P.M.
    Protein drink: 2 glasses milk, ½ cup nonfat milk solids, one egg, ½ cup ice cream. Mix in a blender.

I designed this diet for the individual who either works or is a student. You can rearrange the mealtimes to suit your own schedule, as long as you keep two and a half to three hours between them. Here are a few additional suggestions that should help you gain weight rapidly:

1. Take your own lunch to work. Make sandwiches of roast beef, meat loaf, ground beef, tuna, liverwurst, chicken, turkey, ham, egg, peanut butter or cheese.

2. Use only 100% whole wheat (stone ground is the best), rye, or pumpernickel.

3. If you get hungry between meals, eat cashews. These nuts supply protein, fat and additional calories.

4. Dried fruits are also high in calories and provide extra vitamins and minerals.

5. Use mayonnaise, oil and salad dressings whenever possible with sandwiches, salads and vegetables.

6. Have an extra protein drink on workout days.

7. Plan a definite eating schedule. The body thrives on regularity. Never skip a meal or a snack.

8. Here are three good weight-gaining snacks using cottage cheese:

(A) Cottage cheese (½ pint) with can of tuna, avocado.

(B) Cottage cheese, mixed with fresh or canned fruit.

(C) Cottage cheese, mixed with a bag of cashew nuts.

9. To help maintain your water balance while training, squeeze the juice of one or two lemons into a quart of warm water, add three tablespoons of honey, and shake until it is thoroughly mixed. Sip this drink between exercises during your work-out to replace lost water.

10. A good appetite stimulant is two ounces of red wine mixed with an egg yolk, to drink about half an hour before a meal.

11. A terrific muscle-building dish is my own special version of the "muscle-burger":

      1 pound ground sirloin
      3 whole eggs
      8 Wheat Thin whole wheat crackers (or
         saltines)
      chopped green onions

Using a fork, mix the eggs with the meat in a
large bowl. Crush the crackers up into small
crumbs and add along with the chopped onions.
Keep stirring until the mixture becomes semi-
thick. Cook as you would a regular hambur-
ger—do not overcook.

Types of Exercises

You will use three general types of exercises in developing your body:

1. Upper-body exercises—to build up the arms,
chest, shoulders and back muscles.

2. Lower-body exercises—to build up the thighs
and calves and strengthen the legs and hips.

3. Abdominal exercises—to tighten, tone and muscularize the waist and improve the posture.

You should look at your body in a mirror and divide
it into these three areas—the upper body, the middle
body and the lower body. Each part is as important as
the others. A lot of people think they should work only
on their chest and arms. This is wrong. Each part
needs as much attention as the other two. You need
the abdominals to contain the vital organs and tie the
body together; you need the lower back for lifting
things; you need the legs, the calves, the whole upper
body. Each muscle in the body is important. The
calves count as much as the biceps. People lose big
contests for not having good calves. People have even
lost competitions because of weak forearms. So you
divide your body into the three areas, be aware of
them, and train them with equal enthusiasm.

No matter what your individual development problems may be, you will be doing exercises for all three
areas. If you are soft and flabby and need to lose
weight, obviously you will have to do more of the
abdominal exercises and follow a low-carbohydrate re-
duced-calorie diet. If you are underweight, you should

do mostly upper- and lower-body exercises, and follow a high-protein high-calorie diet. If your weight is about normal, then you can combine all three exercise groups in a unified program while maintaining a normal, balanced diet with special emphasis on protein foods.

Chapter Two
Laying the Foundation

Freehand Exercise

In the beginning it is advisable for you to lay a solid foundation with what we call "freehand exercises." You can do these exercises without expensive gym equipment. You will need only a few pieces of ordinary furniture and your own body.

I became aware of the value of these non-apparatus exercises the summer before I began seriously working with weights. I was hanging out with bodybuilders and other athletes who went to a lake near Graz and did a one-hour exercise routine, which included 15 to 20 exercises that they just made up as they went along. They would look for a tree where they could hang on to the branches and do reverse-grip chin-ups or regular wide-grip chin-ups; they would do push-ups or handstand push-ups or regular push-ups with elevated feet; they would do leg raises and sit-ups. I started working out with them and discovered after a couple of weeks that my body was toned and in better condition than it had ever been.

Freehand exercises have a tonic effect on the muscles and internal organs. They gently tone up the circulatory system and are beneficial in safeguarding the general health of the body. Advanced freehand exercises shape and muscularize the body in a unique way; all the world's best-built men include them in their workouts. Freehand exercises help build muscle size,

174

give definition, and create the kind of muscle contour that gives the body the look of a sculptured Greek god.

Most of the top professional bodybuilders I have either observed or talked to during my career have used the freehand exercise program in one way or another. Some of them used it before they started training with weights, others have continued to use it into their professional lives. It is a routine they get into on the days they don't feel like training with weights or when they are traveling and unable to get to a gym.

Freehand exercises are the perfect way to begin bodybuilding. They will give you the feeling for the first time of having a "pump" in your muscles—as when you do a lot of push-ups and you get a feeling of having blood suddenly rushing into your pectoral muscles. The feeling, called the pump, should be used to tune your body.

I'm going to outline a beginning program that will get you in shape. This is not a sissy program. Let's say your body weight is 150 pounds: you can use the 150 pounds for resistance training. Certain exercises you can do, such as push-ups, give you the same results you'd get from doing a bench press with 150 pounds of heavy steel plates. Doing a handstand push-up is equivalent to doing a press behind the neck or a standing military press. Or if you put a broomstick across two chairs and do pull-ups with a straight body, the effect is the same as bent-over rowing.

These first exercises can be done at home without any expensive equipment. In the beginning you don't need it. You should lay a foundation by stimulating the muscles, tuning the whole body in to resistance training using your own body weight. And after you've accomplished that and feel good about it—which should take from two to six months, depending on your initial condition and your rate of progess—you can safely go into weight training in the gym.

Starting Your Exercise Program

Most people, because of work or school, find it more convenient to exercise in the late afternoon or evening. Your own schedule may dictate that you exercise at some other time—perhaps in the early morning before you go to work. You can make good progess regardless of when you train. I have discovered that I am not the strongest in the morning, but in the morning my body recuperates best, my mind isn't preoccupied, and I can pay the most attention to what I'm doing. So I work out first thing in the morning, from nine to eleven, before I do anything else.

There are two simple rules you should observe:

1. The best time to exercise is about one hour before you eat or two hours after you have eaten a full meal.

2. Try to eat something about two hours before exercising so your energy level will be high.

One mistake many people make is trying to throw two things together, namely food intake and training. They think, "It's lunch break, I'll go eat and then I'll train quickly." But it doesn't work like that. Immediately after you eat, your stomach needs a lot of blood to digest the food. So your working blood supply goes to the stomach. The result of exercising too soon will be poor digestion of your food. I advise never to train immediately before a meal or right after one. In either case it's bad. You should have at least a half to three quarters of an hour for letting your body come down from exercise, and at least three quarters of an hour to an hour for digestion.

Otherwise, there is no "best" time for training. If you work from nine to five you may find it stimulating to get up at six and put in an hour working out before breakfast. A lot of the top bodybuilders who are in business do that. Two perfect examples are Bill Pearl and Reg Park, guys who work out from five to seven A.M. They even trained for the Mr. Universe contest early in the morning, doing squats with 400 and 500 pounds. These are morning people, and they feel morning training is the best for them. There are other people who work best at night. They have to sit down and meditate a little bit to get everything that happened during the day out of their heads and then they get into weight training. They feel perfectly fine working out from ten to twelve at night. It's a personal matter. Through experimentation you must find your own ideal time.

Clothing

What you wear to train in depends on weather conditions. You should be comfortable. If the weather is warm, as it is in California, you should wear tank tops and shorts. Even in cold weather, your clothes should be comfortable—always comfortable, always loose. If you wear two sweatshirts, they should be loose enough to allow you to move without feeling restricted. Try to get clothes that absorb sweat. Cotton is best; polyester and artificial fibers don't absorb as well. A lot of people work out in nylon because they want to look slick. If you start worrying about how your clothes look while you're in training, then you're already training for the wrong reason. You only have to look at your face while you're training and see the sweating and grimacing to realize it's not appealing anyway and that you might as well forget about fashionable gym clothes.

There are times when you want to really sweat and lose weight. Then, you should wear numerous layers of clothes. If your reason for training is to lose weight, and not to build your biceps, calves, or thighs, you should wear things like a rubber reducing belt around your waist, and heavy sweat clothes.

Personally, I prefer to train in as few clothes as possible so I can see my faults. I try to see the specific areas that have fallen behind or that I've neglected. I like to expose them so I have to look at them all the time. For instance, in the beginning my calves were underdeveloped. When I understood how really weak they were, I cut the bottoms off my pants so everybody would see. And that made me eager to train hard and build them up. Most guys in the gym do the opposite. They hide their weak points, which is totally wrong. Before competition I would always walk into the gym to train with no shirt on. Why? Because the instant I sat down I'd see my stomach and say, "Wait a minute, Arnold, you can't go into a contest with a stomach like that, with so much fat on it you get wrinkles." So I would train my waist harder and stay on my diet. It's very important that you expose your weaknesses, that you constantly point them up to yourself. Let the mirror be your reminder.

Breathing

Breathing properly is essential to your health. It's something you should learn from the first movement of your first exercise. If you breathe incorrectly, it could have a bad effect on your lungs and heart. The correct way to breathe when you train is to exhale each time you have some kind of resistance. Let's say you're doing a push-up. When you press your body up from the floor you should breathe out. Remember that one rule: as soon as there is any strain on your body you should breathe out. The time to inhale is when you let yourself down, when your body is under the least amount of pressure.

You should always have plenty of oxygen when you train. This is one reason I prefer to train outdoors whenever possible. Oxygen keeps your energy level up and lets you train longer and harder without exhaustion. If you're training inside, sometimes you have to help your body get the oxygen by taking a lot of vitamin E. But if you have the opportunity, it's best to exercise outside and get the oxygen naturally. Even when I spend most of my time in a gym working out, I try to run, swim and do stretching movements outside in the fresh air. In fact, this first set of exercises, the freehand exercises, could be done outdoors anywhere, even on a porch or balcony.

PUSH-UPS—The first freehand exercise is the push-up. This is an excellent exercise for the chest, shoulders and the back of the arms (triceps). Push-ups are familiar to almost everyone, but most people do them wrong. There is something I want to stress in the beginning: Do not let your ego get in the way of your progess. Perhaps somebody told you you should do 20 or 50 push-ups. Put it out of your mind. Just remember

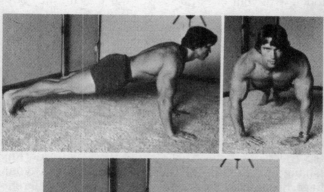

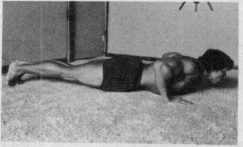

this: The important thing is to do the exercise correctly; that counts for everything. That's why I introduced the basic exercises first, because if you start doing the basic freehand, or non-apparatus, exercises without any problems and without cheating, then you'll go on into weight training without cheating. Right now is the time to catch and correct yourself. You should train only for yourself. If you can do only one push-up but you do it right, that's fine. I'm positive that a week later you'll be able to do three, then six and eventually ten.

Place your hands approximately shoulder width apart. Hold your body perfectly straight and exhale as you push your body up until your arms are straight. Pause. Inhale as you lower your body to the floor, allowing only your chest to touch. Your stomach should still be an inch or two off the floor when you touch with your chest, because your toes lift the body up a bit.

The most important thing is not to touch the floor with your stomach, your head, or your knees, and to press up until your arms are locked straight. You should do it with a steady movement, like a piston, up and down, up and down. And always do full repetitions. The muscle that will get the most from this exercise is the pectoral muscle, the whole pectoral muscle. You will feel blood rushing into this area. But it's not merely the pectoral muscle that pushes up the body; the triceps and the front deltoid work with it. (I'm talking just about the normal push-up with your fingertips toward the front. Later you can use different hand positions to stimulate different muscle areas. For instance, if you start turning the hands toward the inside it will go more into the triceps and deltoid area, less to the pecs.)

Don't worry about the sets and repetitions in the beginning. Within a few weeks, you should work up to a total of 50 repetitions. You can do 10 five times, or 5 ten times. Just pick a certain number of repetitions and *remember to observe the strict form.* If you're athletically talented and have no problem doing 50, then you should go to 100. The number depends on the person, but you should give yourself a nice workout. Some guys struggle with 10 repetitions. Others who do 50 easily should go further, maybe two or three sets of 50. But basically I would start at 50 push-ups a day and work your way up slowly.

If you can do a lot of repetitions easily and you want to get more resistance, elevate your feet, using a chair at first, then a table.

DIPS BETWEEN CHAIRS—Take two chairs that are strong enough to hold your body weight and place them approximately shoulder width apart, back to back, the backs parallel. Take hold of each chair as shown in photo. Bend your legs at the knees, finding a stable way of holding yourself balanced so you don't fall forward, and push your body up until your arms are locked straight. Let your body come down as slowly as you can and try to touch your front deltoids on the chair backs. Then slowly press your body weight up again. Keep your legs bent. Exhale as you push up, inhale as you let your body down. Go up and down evenly but slowly. Look directly ahead during the movements and try to keep your body as straight as possible.

This is a triceps and pectoral and deltoid exercise. Some people lean forward too much so it becomes a strict pectoral exercise, which you've had with push-ups. It should be fifty percent in the triceps, forty percent in the deltoids and ten percent in the shoulders. You should always give it the full repetition. Go all the way down and all the way up. That's a must in the beginning of the workout. The more fully you do the repetition, the more fully your muscle is developed. The reason some bodybuilders develop short pectorals, short biceps, short triceps is that they don't do full movements.

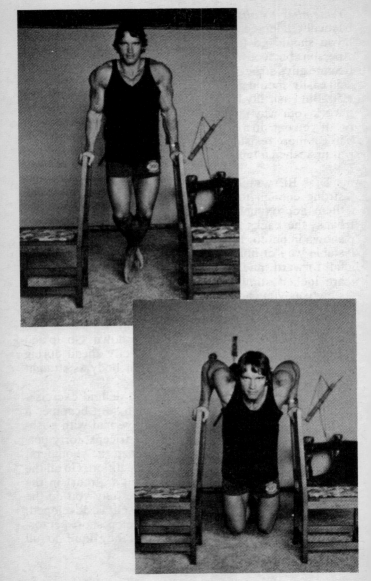

You may find this exercise difficult in the beginning, but work at it until you can do 50 repetitions. Again, how you arrive at 50 doesn't matter in the first month. After you get into it and can accomplish a certain number of repetitions easily, you should strive to do five sets of 20. You can't work too much, that's for sure. However, it's very important not to cheat. Don't get hung up on the number of repetitions; just get hung up on strict form. It would be better for your body to do 5 *perfect* dips than to do 50 sloppy ones. I'm going to repeat that idea over and over throughout this book: Doing exercises correctly, perfectly, doing full movements, is the most important thing in bodybuilding.

ROWING BETWEEN CHAIRS—This exercise is extremely good for tuning up the back muscles—the upper back, the center back, the outside back and the latissimus. Place two chairs approximately five feet apart and put a broomstick across the backs. Lie on the floor between the chairs and grip the broomstick,

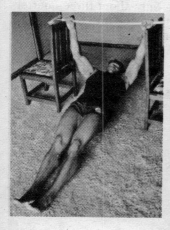
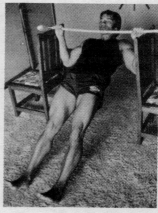

as you see me doing in the photograph. Then, keeping
your heels on the floor, pull yourself all the way up to
the broomstick and let yourself slowly down again.
Hold your body absolutely straight, as with push-ups.
The only part that should move is your arms. Pull the
broomstick in to your chest area, making it touch each
time.

Do as many repetitions as you can in the beginning
and work up to a total of at least 50.

BENT-LEG SIT-UPS—This is a terrific abdominal
conditioner, working mostly to tighten the upper abdomen. Put your feet under a piece of furniture, a bed or
a couch, and bend your legs at a 45-degree angle. Sit-
ups are more beneficial when done with the legs bent
because this puts all of the stress on the front abdominal muscles, thus eliminating any assistance from the
hip flexors, which occurs when the legs are straight.
Hold your hands in front of your waist with your
fingers knit together and go up and down. It is not
necessary to lie back fully—only about three-quarters
of the way—but the movement should be very smooth
and rhythmical. With abdominals all you need is contraction. It's actually one of the few sets of muscles we
don't give a full movement. We want to flex the muscles, to compress them.

Do 100 repetitions, two sets of 50. If you feel comfortable doing 100 you can try 150 or 200.

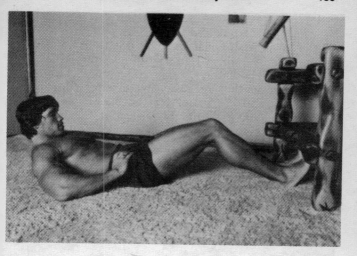

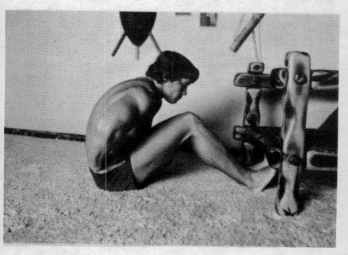

BENT LEG RAISES—Bent leg raises warm up the muscles of the trunk and lower back and burn the fat off the lower abdominal area. Sit-ups train the upper abdominals, the upper two rows, and leg raises work on the lower abdominals. I suggest leg raises with bent knees because they're easier, you can get in more repetitions, and it's better for the back. Lie on the floor with your legs straight out, your hands under your buttocks, and your chin on your chest (this posi-

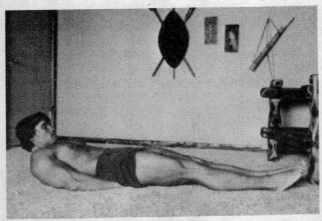

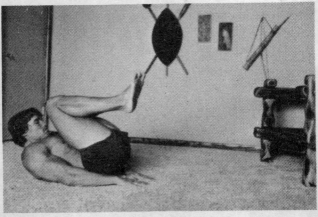

tion of the head and neck causes your abdominals to flex when you are in a prone position); then pull your knees all the way into your chest area.

Remember the rule about breathing—exhale as you bring up your legs, inhale as you lower them. Do as many repetitions as you can, so the flexing and extending can burn the fat off your midsection and tighten up those muscles. In this exercise the amount of resistence is not nearly as important as how many repetitions you do.

Try to do a minimum of 50 repetitions.

BENT-OVER TWISTS—Twists are for the obliques, those muscles at the sides of the waist, and for the lower back. They're a great exercise for trimming off

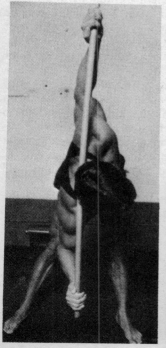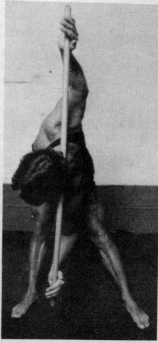

excess fat. I suggest you do them in the following manner: Take a broomstick and put it behind your neck, gripping it wide with your hands. Hold your legs stiff, your feet about shoulder width apart, and bend forward until your upper body is at a 45-degree angle to your legs (as in photo). Now twist your body in half-circular motions, bringing the ends of the stick down to touch your feet, alternating right and left, right and left. You'll feel this one start to burn immediately.

As with leg raises and sit-ups, it's the number of repetitions here that really counts. Go for at least 50 reps and work up.

Remember what I said about cheating. Just to remind myself, I slip in an extra rep or two. Try it. It'll make you feel better about your program.

DEEP KNEE BENDS (SQUATS)—Squats will build up your thighs and strengthen your hips. They can be done in different ways. One way is to stand with your heels on a book, go all the way down, and come all the way up. The other is to stand flatfooted on the floor and go all the way up and down. I suggest you use a book, as you see me doing in the photo. Stand with your feet 12 to 15 inches apart and place your hands on your hips. Squat down until your thighs are parallel to the floor, then raise yourself slowly up again. Remember to keep your body upright and your back straight throughout the exercise. Breathe deeply—inhaling as you squat, exhaling as you come back up—and hold your chest high and square. One method of making the repetitions smooth and even is to choose a point on the wall and look at it as you do the exercise.

Do 50 to 70 repetitions.

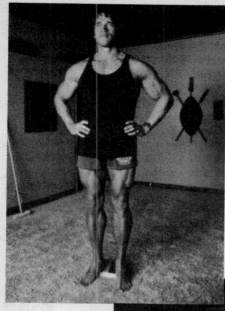

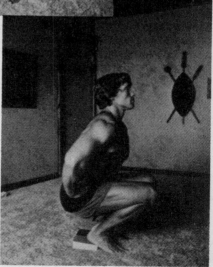

CALF RAISES—I think the calf is the most beautiful muscle in the body. Certainly the calves are the prime muscles of the leg. Think for a minute, if you saw a man at the beach with big muscular thighs but scrawny calves, you would say he had bad legs. However, if he had poor thighs but fantastic calves, you would probably say how good his legs were. Unfortunately, the calves are difficult to develop. They are made of dense muscle fibers that must really be bombed to be altered.

You should do calf raises standing on a book, only now your toes should be elevated so they are higher than your heels. Hold the back of a chair lightly for balance. Your feet should be parallel and a few inches apart. Lower your heels to the floor, stretching the calf muscle, and then raise all the way up on your toes. This develops the whole calf.

Do at least 50 repetitions.

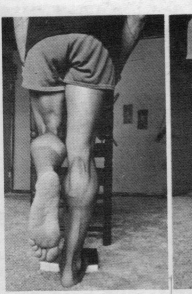
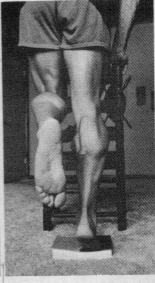

CLOSE-GRIP BICEPS CHINS—This is probably the only exercise you can do without gym equipment to build impressive biceps. However, you will need a chinning bar. You can buy an inexpensive bar that fits between doorjambs. Take an underhand grip (palms facing toward your body) on the chinning bar, with the hands about 12 inches apart. Starting with your arms straight, pull up until your chin is over the bar and your biceps are fully contracted. Lower your body slowly until your arms are straight. Chin-ups are tough when they're done right, but they will really pack inches onto your biceps. Go all the way down and all the way up, making full movements. Stretch when you reach the bottom and pull all the way up to the chin. Do not kick with your legs to put you that last few inches to the top. This robs you of the benefits of the exercise.

Do as many repetitions as you can, trying for a total of 30.

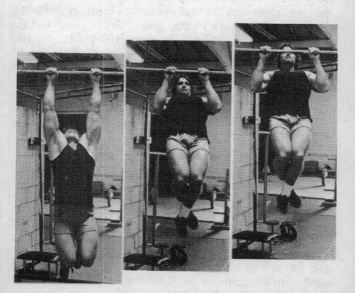

After the Workout—Jogging and Swimming

Practice these exercises throughout the entire body-building program. They accustom the body to its new weight and configuration and help you avoid becoming "musclebound."

Bodybuilding can stiffen the body. It happens this way: Blood rushes into the muscle, gives you a pump, and makes you stiff. To counteract and correct this you should try something different from the exercises you do in the gym. Jogging and swimming will satisfy these needs by helping to stretch and lengthen your muscles and eliminate the danger of becoming "musclebound."

JOGGING—There are different kinds of jogging. Running around the block is okay, but I would suggest something more imaginative, such as cross-country running, which is running up and down hills, jumping over trees, and other things that really get the body moving. (Jumping on and off curbs, dodging between parking meters and cars can give a similar result). Also interval training, where you sprint 100 yards, jog 100 yards, sprint 100 yards, will get the heart working and the blood flowing. Vary the running so that you don't get stale. Sometimes you're forced to jog indoors, where you just stay in one place and imitate running to get your heart going. You should do this only when you're traveling or on winter days when it's impossible for you to go outside.

SWIMMING—Swimming is a highly effective muscle toner. The smooth reach and follow-through of swimming lengthens your muscles and keeps them flexible. I love swimming and I've been doing it almost daily for the last 15 years. Swimming is one of those activities that force you to use your muscles in such a way that they flow together and make your body work as a total, integrated unit. It is even more beneficial if you can swim outdoors in the sunshine and fresh air.

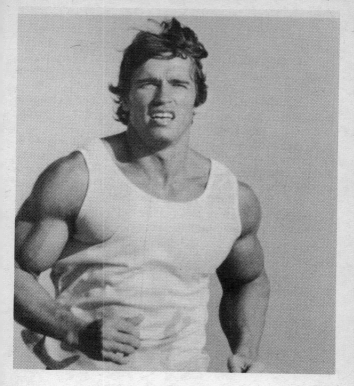

Some Hints about Training

1. Give your full concentration to each exercise. Feel what the exercise does to your muscles as you move.

2. Good form is more important than the number of repetitions. Add more resistance as you get stronger, but never at the expense of good exercise form.

3. After your workout stand in front of a mirror and check your body. Do a few poses. Make an honest assessment of your progress.

4. Maintain a positive mental attitude at all times.

5. You must eat well and get adequate sleep when you are on a serious bodybuilding program. You need eight to nine hours of sound, restful sleep every night. Mending and growth take place during these periods of rest. If for some reason you miss your quota of sleep, take a half-hour to one-hour nap after you get home from work. This will refresh you, help you recuperate more fully, and speed your progress.

6. Anything worth doing at all is worth doing well. Put your heart and soul into your training, diet and sleep programs. Success in bodybuilding could be a key to other successes. It has been for me. I believe you can do anything you want—build a great body, obtain wealth, be a success in life—if you want it badly enough and are willing to work for it with all your heart.

Chapter Three
Progressive Resistance Weight Training

Choosing Your Gym

You'll be doing at least a one-hour workout in the beginning, and eventually a two-hour workout, so it's important that you choose a place where you feel one hundred percent comfortable and where you will be inspired to do hard work.

In the last fourteen years I've found some gymnasiums I've felt incredibly good in—where I immediately got wonderful vibrations and a sudden flow of energy because of the way they looked—and other gymnasiums that depressed me as soon as I walked through the door. I especially don't like the kind of gym that gives a sense of relaxation.

One consideration in evaluating a gym is who works out there. It helps if a lot of bodybuilders are training for competition. That's the kind of atmosphere you want. You can relate to these people and let them guide you in attaining the proper workout spirit. I personally choose the places with heavy wheels and cables and machines, heavy-duty stuff that looks like torture equipment. That kind of gym gives me the incentive to do a serious workout. I've found that, generally speaking, home gyms can have a negative effect on concentrated training. Your kitchen and living room are too close. You find yourself thinking,

"Should I do another set or should I watch television?"
There are too many temptations. But if you make the
commitment of traveling to the gym for half an hour,
you will most likely decide that you're going to put in
some work so you won't have gone there for nothing.

The gymnasium you choose should have good venti-
lation. Next to your mental attitude, plentiful oxygen
is actually the most important thing while you're training. Without an adequate oxygen supply you will tire
easily and be unable to handle a vigorous one- or two-
hour workout.

The gym should be cool—if it's too hot you will
grow languid and feel your strength has been sapped.
Preferably you should get fresh air, not air-conditioned
air. That's why I like World's Gym in Santa Monica;
it's close to the beach and fresh ocean air, which I
think gives you a little bit more energy than regular air.
If you have the chance to work outdoors (as I sometimes do when I go to the outdoor weight-lifting platform at Venice Beach) do so. Working out in the sun
tightens your skin and gives you a good color. Which
in turn adds a great deal to the way you feel about your
body.

Mental Attitude

Do not underestimate the part your attitude plays in
bodybuilding. Mental strain and worry can drain the
body and adversely affect both your workouts and
muscular growth. A good positive mental attitude
ought to go beyond the gym. It should extend to your
eating habits, your sleeping habits, and the way you
conduct your life in general.

Use the time on the way to the gym to outline some
immediate goals for yourself, to decide what you want
to accomplish in this particular workout session. Don't
just go to the gym and say, "Oh, no, another workout." Your attitude should be: "Okay, this is another

training session, and today instead of a 100-pound bench press I'll do 105 pounds. I feel stronger today; I can do it. I can do more chin-ups. I can do more sit-ups."

You should set goals for yourself that turn you on and make you eager to go in and do bench presses, or squats, or barbell curls. Have a definite reason for wanting to do bench presses. Not just because you want to look better next year. That is a long-range goal, which is very important—but you should also be setting little short-range goals all the time. For example, tell yourself that tomorrow morning you want to get a good pump in the pectoral muscles. Or, yesterday you saw a picture of a bodybuilder whose waist was 29 inches, and you would like to have really good abdominals, so today you'll do more repetitions: by next Monday you ought to be half an inch smaller in the waist. These little goals are fantastic. They've helped me a lot. Of course I always said I wanted to be Mr. Universe or Mr. Olympia. But that was long-range thinking. In addition I always had day-to-day goals, which included measurement increases of a quarter of an inch, two or three more repetitions, and five pounds of added weight on the barbell.

The Warm-up Period

Very few people have jobs that require much physical exertion. You sit at a desk. You move a lot without being conscious of your muscles. So when it comes time to exercise, it's important to let your body warm up. You can use that period to tune in mentally as well as physically.

Give your body a chance to adjust to the new activity. It's a way of saying to the body, "I'm giving you a warm-up now, take your time, fall into it easily. In a few minutes I'm going to hit you hard!" That should be your attitude toward your muscles. Do a warm-up of push-ups, pull-downs, squats with no weights, circling your arms around and a series of stretching movements.

I always warm up the specific body parts I want to train. For example, for the shoulders and arms I take a 30- or 40-pound weight, which is really light, and do twenty or thirty repetitions to get a lot of blood into the area. I do curls with light weights then some triceps bench presses and behind-the-neck presses to warm up the elbow area and the shoulder joints and loosen up my shoulders and arms. I don't try to build the muscle, I only get the blood flowing. The danger of not warming up and preparing your body for heavier resistance training is that you may tear your muscles and get aches that will discourage you from continuing.

When I was training for contests, I'd sometimes be so psyched up mentally I thought I didn't need a warm-up. I'd go directly into a heavy workout. Without fail, I'd pull muscles needlessly and set myself back two or three months.

Training Partner

I have found that the best way to get great workouts is to have an enthusiastic training partner. You'll be amazed at how much harder and faster you can work when you have someone to work out with. A good training partner pushes you to handle more poundage and gives you the incentive to grind out more reps per set with a minimum of rest pauses in between (which is real quality training). Workouts are more fun with a partner as well as more competitive. On those days when you feel lazy, your partner pushes you to keep working hard, and you end up with a good workout instead of an incomplete one.

Your partner should be someone you like and respect, someone you want to respect you. You can have little competitions. You say to him, "I feel good, today. I'm going to put 200 pounds in the bar and do ten repetitions instead of eight." And he says, "If you do ten I'll do twelve." You challenge each other and yourselves. You bet a mug of beer or a bottle of wine. All these little gimmicks, as childish as they may sound, make a workout exciting, interesting and much more rewarding.

The Basic Exercises

Let me say a word about the ten exercises in this chapter. They are geared for the major muscle groups—not for little muscle groups. They are basic to the development of the major areas of your body. They will give you the foundation and mass you'll need for later refinement. You must use them in the beginning, and you must continue to use them as you progress. The first exercise, the *bench press,* is absolutely necessary for a big chest. There is no exercise to replace it. I started doing the bench press when I was fifteen and I've been doing it now for fourteen years.

These exercises are to be done three times a week, with one day between workouts for mending and setting. Basically, the theory is simple. In the beginning you will be training your whole body in one day. This should be followed by a rest day because it takes forty-eight hours for the muscles to recuperate, to rebuild to their normal size and grow bigger. If you trained a muscle every day it would slowly deteriorate—you would be just tearing it down and not rebuilding it. Also, you need forty-eight hours to let the joints recuperate. Since, in the beginning, you will do basic movements for every muscle at each workout, you need a day of rest between your sessions in the gym.

The basic exercises will appear throughout the entire training program. There are no alternatives to these exercises. For example, every bodybuilder has to do squats from the time he starts until he finishes.

You can't build your legs without the squat. The detail stuff that gives you more definition is fine, but the basic thigh muscle can only be developed and maintained by doing heavy squats. If you try to get away from them the size of the muscle will go down. Barbell curls, triceps extensions behind the neck, calf raises, sit-ups are the same—you can't get around them. Basic exercises work directly on the muscle. You fall into a groove and don't even have to think about anything except the pump and the form of the exercise. With the complicated exercises, you have to concentrate all your thought on the exercise and not the muscle. I think the reason some bodybuilders use delicate exercises, which I call chicken exercises, is that they don't feel confident with the basic movements or with themselves. The bench press seems so simple, they think they should do something more complicated. But you can't use as much weight when you make the exercise difficult, so it takes away from the meaning of heavy training.

It all goes back to mental attitude, back to being confident in your program. You have to believe that sooner or later you will achieve the body you want. You won't waste your time searching for programs, exotic food supplements and "secret" exercises. There are no "secret" exercises in bodybuilding. The secret is not what exercises to do but how to do them.

Sets and Repetitions

In the beginning—unless stated otherwise in the specific exercise—I would suggest doing three sets of 8 to 10 repetitions of each exercise. Thirty sets altogether should be done in 45 minutes, or at most, an hour. This allows for a 30-second rest period between sets.

1. BENCH PRESS—This is the number-one exercise for increasing the mass of the upper body, especially

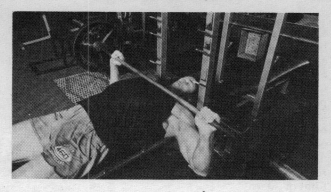

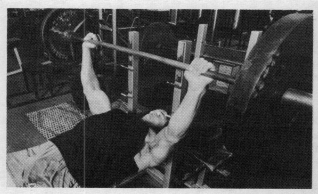

the pectoral muscles. Lie down on the exercise bench
with your feet approximately 18 inches apart for support. Using a fairly wide grip (as in photo) lower the
barbell until it touches your chest about nipple level
and then ram it back up overhead. Lock your elbows
at the top. Inhale deeply on the way down, exhale
going up. Use the add-weight system (add a small
amount of weight at the beginning of each set) for five
sets (8, 8, 6, 6, 6 reps respectively).

2. WIDE-GRIP CHINS—These chins widen the lats and work on the entire shoulder girdle. Many top bodybuilders have built great upper backs with this exercise alone. It primarily develops the upper and outer regions of the lats and spreads the scapula, making it easier to widen the lats. Using a wide grip (see photo), pull yourself up until your chin is over the bar; lower the body slowly and give the lats a good stretch on the way down. I prefer 10 reps, and sometimes I add weight by placing a dumbbell between my legs for a few sets of 6 to 8 reps. You may not be able to do 10 reps. In that case do as many as you can, aiming for a total of 30.

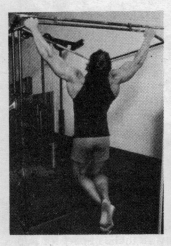

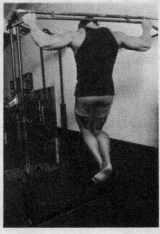

3. MILITARY PRESS—The military press is for the deltoid muscles. The front deltoid is the biggest muscle here and a pressing movement with a barbell is basic to its development. Your grip on the bar should be about 5 inches wider than your shoulders. Sitting with your feet approximately a foot apart, lift the barbell from the floor to the chest area, which is called cleaning the weight; then in a second movement press it slowly and smoothly over your head and lock your elbows. This exercise can also be performed from a standing position; however, I prefer the sitting version because it eliminates excessive strain on the lower back. I would strongly recommend that you use a sturdy lifting belt. Again, you can use the add-weight principle.

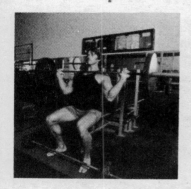

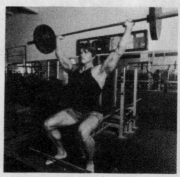

4. BARBELL CURL—I believe in basic moves, and the standing barbell curl couldn't be more basic for building the biceps. At first, I suggest you take a medium-wide grip (approximately shoulder-width) on the bar to hit the bicep directly, although later on you can vary the grip to the degree that you personally feel the greatest results. As with all exercises, start with a weight that becomes progressively more difficult to lift after about the fifth rep. This strain rams the blood into the biceps. Remember, this is a power-building as well as a muscle-building exercise so don't be afraid to handle the poundage. Only your forearms should move. Keep your elbows stationary. If you allow them to move, the deltoids will do the work and you will not get 100% bicep action.

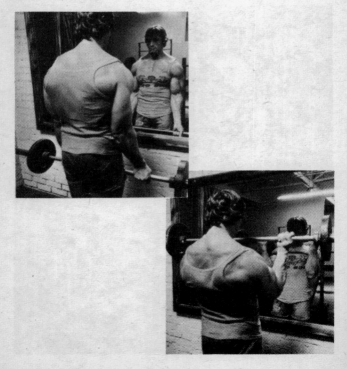

5. FRENCH PRESS—Grip the bar with your hands approximately 10 inches apart and lift it over your head. Keep your upper arm in a stationary position close to the sides of your head. Let the weight slowly down behind your head. Then press the weight slowly back to the starting position. Do not allow your upper arms to move.

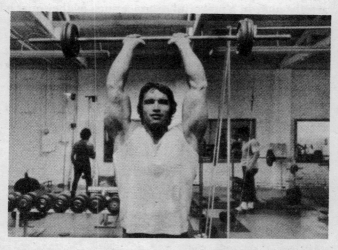

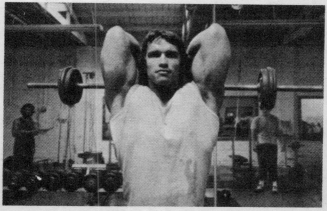

6. SQUATS, WEIGHT BEHIND THE NECK—Squats will develop your thighs, strengthen your heart and lungs, and generally improve your circulation. It is better to do this exercise with the aid of a squat rack so you can use heavy weight. Holding the weight on the back of your shoulders, with your feet either flat on the floor or with the heels elevated by one-inch blocks, keep your upper body straight and lower yourself into a full squat. In a powerful exercise such as the squat it is essential to remember the rules about breathing. Inhale deeply on the way down, exhale while coming up. I would recommend that you do the squat in front of a mirror so you can observe your form and always keep the weight parallel and your upper body as straight as possible. One word of caution: If you do squats crooked you leave yourself open to serious injury in the lumbar region.

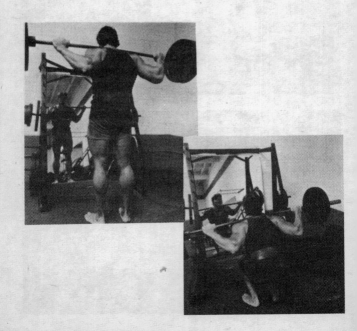

7. LEG CURL—I do leg curls on the leg curl machine. No exercise works more directly on the backs of the thighs, the leg biceps. Lie on your stomach on the bench of the machine, hook your heels under the lever bar, then, holding the sides of the bench, pull the weight toward your buttocks. Bring your heels as far forward as you can, then lower the weight slowly. Let it go all the way down to give your muscles a long stretch. Be sure that your legs move only from the knees down. Do not allow your hips to help lift the

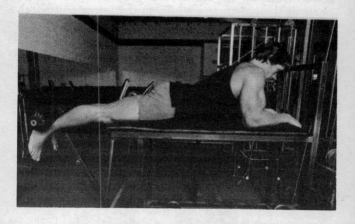

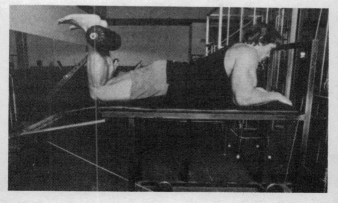

weight. If you do, the curls will be far less effective. It is important to let the legs go straight, then to curl the weight up as far as possible. If a leg curl machine is not available, you can improvise by placing a dumbbell between your feet as you lie prone on a flat bench, and then curl the weight up. Naturally, the curl machine is best because of its constant leverage and resistance.

8. CALF RAISES ON CALF MACHINE—Standing calf raises work on the inside, outside, lower and upper parts of the calves to give them thickness and width. The normal position is to stand on the wooden block at the base of the machine, with your toes pointed straight forward. Situate your shoulders under the

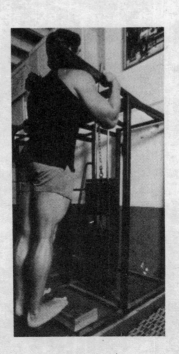

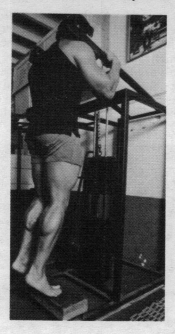

padded bars, as in the photograph, and lift as high as you can on your toes. Let yourself down slowly, allowing your heels to drop as far below the platform as they will. You should feel the stretch in your calves until it hurts. The most common mistake people make is putting on so much weight they cannot observe the strict form. When the weight gets so heavy it is difficult to get all the reps out, some people will bend their knees and use their thighs to complete the exercise. This is wrong. The right way to do the exercise and get the best results is to keep the knees locked, let the heels down as far as possible, and go up until the calf is cramped.

Because the calf is a difficult muscle, you should do five sets of 15 reps.

9. SIT-UPS WITH LEGS BENT—The stomach is the turbine of the torso. We should be concerned about it for both health and appearance. It is the center, the area from which we draw our life forces. In addition, the abdominals are the muscles the judges look at first in a physique contest. Without good solid abs you can never have a chance at winning trophies. We've discussed this exercise in the previous chapter. If you've

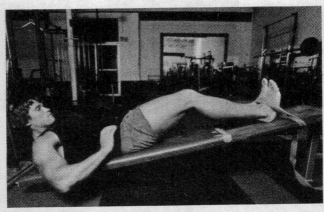

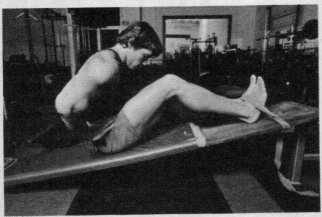

done it properly, you should have noticed that your waist is trimmer by inches, your posture is 100% better, and your digestion and elimination are improved. To add resistance you can do the sit-ups on a slant board, as shown in photo.

Do three sets of 50.

10. WRIST CURL—Wrist curls work on the flexors of the forearm and also increase finger strength. The forearm muscles should not be neglected. They are as important as the muscles in the shoulders and lats and

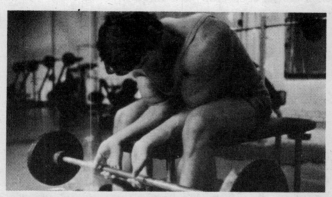

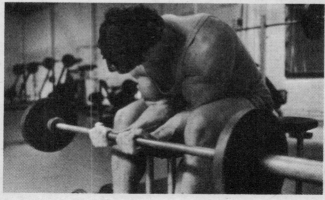

calves. I prefer doing the curls in a sitting position, resting the back of my forearms on the bench and holding the barbell in a close grip. It is very important to keep your elbows together. To be sure that the elbows always stay in a close position, I lock them between my knees (refer to picture). Moving only your wrist, curl the weight up until your forearm is fully contracted. Allow the weight to go down slowly, then at the bottom let the bar roll out on your extended fingers. The forearm, like the calf, is a hard muscle to reach. Do as many full reps as you can, then continue with partial reps until your forearm is tight and burning. Don't worry about pain; it means growth.

Muscle Awareness

Certain areas of your body will get sore during training. I've already mentioned that the first time I worked out I couldn't walk or lift anything for days afterward. You'll have experiences like that, and you should remember them as being beautiful. Memorize those feelings, remember why they happened. "Because of a standing press my deltoid was sore from the collarbone to the biceps." This puts you in touch with your body; in the future when you do standing presses you'll know what to concentrate on. This is only the beginning of what I call muscle awareness. You should use it and push yourself to the point at which you feel your mind is actually in your muscle. Eventually you'll find that if you concentrate hard enough you will be able to send blood to a particular muscle just by thinking about it. So memorize the soreness and use it as a reference for concentration.

When you exercise you should be totally aware of the muscle you are working on. You'll be able to borrow power from other areas of your body. When that happens, you'll know you've made the connection between mind and body, mind and muscle.

Words of Caution to the Beginner

Unless you were unusually fit, you should have trained for at least four to six months on the freehand exercise program before going to the gym. This period of "foundation training" is necessary to tune your body for actual weight training. You will never regret the time you invested in it. The worst mistake the average aspiring bodybuilder makes is attempting to do too much. This results in overtraining, no muscle growth, and total discouragement. Follow my instructions and you'll stay on the right path.

You should not favor one muscle or muscle group over another. Perform all exercises with equal energy and enthusiasm. The name of the game is to do as much for each muscle as possible, and to develop the entire body uniformly.

Progress and Advancement

Your rate of progress depends on the goals you've set. If you are training just to get in shape, you can stay with this program for six months. If you want to get into competitive bodybuilding, you will take less time; you'll be giving it more thought and training more seriously, and you may very likely move on to the next program in three months.

Overtraining

Training too much is as bad—if not worse—than not training enough. Somehow you will have to trust your body to tell you when you are overtraining. It lets you know through excessive aches and pains. However, with the kind of program I've given you here I don't think it's possible to overtrain—and you shouldn't misread simple soreness. As I've said before, soreness is a sign that you are reaching the muscles, that they are responding and starting to grow.

Stretching

Stretching is important while you're exercising. When you are first starting, it can be as important as the training program. You should understand how to develop yourself so you don't end up with a clumsy, "musclebound" body. The musclebound body is created by people who only lift weights and flex and contract their muscles, whose only thought is to get muscles. They never go beyond the flexing and contracting to the other movements the muscles need in order to stay supple. Stretching the muscles, making them long and limber, is one of the things that sets off the champion from the guy who is as big as the champion but who doesn't look as good.

As soon as I started doing the stretching exercises my muscles started flowing together, my whole body began looking more symmetrical. My movements became more balletlike, my posing improved, and the way I walked and handled myself was more elegant. My body had more flexibility. It felt better. You can imagine what your body goes through when you do only heavy resistance training and never allow the muscles to straighten out. I've seen musclemen who couldn't bend over and touch their toes any more. They had flexed so much that their tendons had shortened.

I got into stretching movements very late. I had already won the Mr. Universe title twice and had moved to America before someone introduced me to stretching. This was a guy who was into yoga as well as bodybuilding. He told me how important it is for someone doing weight lifting to stretch. I became aware of it when I watched him do yoga and saw how supple and limber he was. I started to analyze what it takes

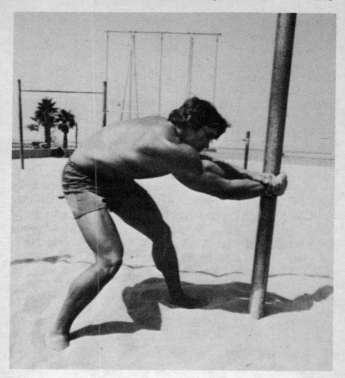

for the body and the muscle to stretch right after an exercise. I devised some stretching exercises I could do after every workout, and it helped me tremendously. You can do the same, taking your cues from your own body and what you feel it needs.

The point of stretching is to elongate the muscle, relax it, and let the blood flow through it, so it should not be done with the same kind of contraction as the exercises that go before. On days you exercise your legs, for example, you can do stretches dancers use: sit on the floor with your legs spread and knees straight and pull your toes as far up toward your body as they will go; or, standing, lift your leg and brace the heel on a table or chair back as high as you can manage without bending your knees. Hold these positions for 30 seconds.

For the back, hang from a chinning bar and let your back stretch (this is also good for the pectorals). For the abdominal area, stand with your hands clasped behind your head and pull the abs till they're firm. Hold positions for about 30 seconds, breathing naturally. You can also grab hold of a bar or machine and pull back with your body, concentrating the stretch wherever it is needed. (See photograph).

This is my personal routine, which I developed according to what I sensed to be my body's needs. You will discover that your own body has its own particular requirements and will find it easy to work out your own routine of stretches to meet them. Just remember: the purpose of stretching is not to continue the workout but to provide a kind of a wind-down.

Chapter Four
Developing the Muscle Groups

Introduction

You ought to be at a point now where you can look at yourself and see incredible changes. You will have trimmed off excess fat, firmed up your muscles, and added a new dimension and symmetry to your body. You should now be able to envision further possibilities for your development.

I find there are two types of people in bodybuilding. One is more interested in doing the exercises properly and in the proper form. He concentrates on handling the weight in full, smooth repetitions. As a result, he builds a symmetrical body. The other kind of guy has his mind geared not so much toward the feeling of the exercise as toward ego satisfaction. He wants to lift a lot of weight. In many cases this person will handle more weight than the person who does the exercises in strict form, but he won't achieve the same results. So remember this: It isn't how much weight you handle but rather how much weight you handle in the correct form that will give you the best body.

Ed Corney and Frank Zane, both former Mr. Universes, and myself are examples of bodybuilders who are more concerned with form than weight. We handle only enough weight to make the exercise challenging, but we do it in strict form. I wasn't always into form over weight. But when I came to America I was forced to go through a lot of changes. Frank Zane beat me in Florida, which taught me I wasn't as perfect as I thought.

I had been beaten before by Chet Yorton, in 1966. But then I felt there was nothing wrong, because he'd been bigger. With Frank Zane it was more disturbing. I came over having won Mr. Universe twice and he had never won anything except Mr. America. He weighed 185, which was 60 pounds less than I weighed. I couldn't figure out *why* he had won. My first thought was that if a big guy lost to a little guy the contest was fixed. It was one of the very few times in my life I ever cried. I cried the whole night after the contest. But I kept thinking about it—what does Zane have that I don't have? I studied photographs of him and came to the conclusion that his muscles were better developed, he had more detail, more quality, more separation, and more muscularity than I did. So I knew what areas I had to work on. I realized that the biggest guy doesn't always win. I started changing my ideas about bigness and started to think about perfection. I had to stop struggling with huge poundages to build mass. What I needed were more repetitions, full repetitions. The more attention I paid to strict form, the closer I brought myself to the perfect body I wanted.

Positive Mental Attitude and Muscle Awareness

Before you begin your workouts sit down for a few moments and think about your body. Let your mind get in touch with your muscles. During the day you probably think about everything except training your body. You shouldn't just hurry to the gym from a business deal and start doing a bench press. Not only will the exercise do you no good, it may actually injure you. The mind doesn't work like that. You should allow it a few minutes to adjust to the idea of training. It is especially valuable now to be aware of your body, mind and muscles, separately and as a single unit. Start with your calves. Feel them, flex them. Work up from there. Flex your thighs, your abdominals; feel the control you have, get in touch mentally with all those body parts—the biceps, the triceps; flex your deltoids, try to flex your latissimus. Get a sense of each body part. Let it register in your mind that your body needs to be trained. Look into the mirror, see how your muscles look, ask yourself how they are coming along. Be honest with yourself. What do you need? And as you do this your mind will change and get tuned in to your body.

The Value of Alternate-Day Training Building and Healing

The reason we split up the exercises is to give 48 hours of rest to the muscles, to allow them to recuperate from injury or soreness. At first we don't want to train the same muscles every day (there are exceptions—abdominals, calves and forearms, which we use every day and must therefore train in a different way. The muscles in the abdomen are vital to almost every body function, the forearms are needed to grip, the calves to walk). In this program we will divide up the week so that we work on three major muscle groups one day and three minor muscle groups the next day.

Your Training Partner

A training partner now becomes a critical matter. He is a person you have to rely on 100%. The further you get into bodybuilding, the more important your partner becomes. For me, he's as important as a business partner—it becomes a marriage. You commit yourself. You don't just train together. You help each other. The times when you don't feel good, the other person lifts up your spirits and your energy level.

The problem with training alone is that you sometimes don't feel strong. You're down physically. For instance, you want to do a bench press with 300 pounds, 8 repetitions, but you're worried that you may not be able to handle the last rep, and this huge weight on your chest could actually kill you. If you have a training partner, he can stand behind you, count out the repetitions, and help you if anything goes wrong. Sometimes the last repetition seems so hard you don't think you can make it. He takes off the pressure by just putting a single finger under the bar and pressing up a little bit. These are called forced reps. They can really count for the pump and muscle growth. Your partner is also there to compliment you continuously. You live off each other's compliments and ego boosting.

You constantly need help in a gymnasium. You need somebody to watch how you are progressing and to suggest changes in your training style. He says, "Listen, I'm still not satisfied with your waist. Maybe you're doing your sit-ups wrong." He can check it out. Also, after a workout you discuss training problems. You can show off to a training partner, have little ongoing competitions. It motivates you to push harder when you can reveal new progress to your partner.

The Four-Day Routine

This routine gives you four days a week in the gym: Monday–Thursday and Tuesday–Friday. during the three days off you should concentrate on swimming, jogging and stretching movements. You should not do any weight resistance training on those days. Break your body in slowly, allowing it at least a month to get accustomed to the new routine.

MONDAY AND THURSDAY PROGRAM

On Mondays and Thursdays we will work on the legs, chest, abdomen.

I always train the chest and the legs together on principle. Because the leg workout takes a lot of heavy breathing, you also train your lungs. While you're squatting you draw in huge amounts of air and expand your chest, so your chest is already warmed up, and you can move on to your chest workout and get a two-shot effect.

You should train abdominals and calves every day.

The Legs—Thighs and Calves

The frontal group of muscles in the thigh are the *extensors*. As a major muscle group, they are often referred to as the *quadriceps*. The longest of these is the *rectus femorus,* which arises from the anterior inferior iliac spine and inserts into the patella. It overlays the *vastus intermedium,* which arises from the femur and inserts into the patella. These two muscles make the central "V"-shaped delineation of the middle front thigh. The formation on the inner thigh is the *vastus medialus,* and the outer thigh muscle is called the *vastus lateralis,* both of which originate at the upper head of the femur and insert into the patella. The muscle group generates great power and is best developed by direct leg extensions and squatting.

Two muscles flex the thigh toward the abdomen. One is fairly short and can be seen around the lateral hip joint. It is the *tensor fascae latae* and arises from the lateral border of the ilium to the lateral fascia of the thigh. The second muscle, the sartorius, is the longest in the body, and runs diagonally across the thigh. The action of these muscles, which elevate and extend the thigh, is not unlike the action of triceps in the upper arm.

While not as showy as the frontal extensors, the thigh *flexors* complete the thigh movement and add tremendously to thigh size. The deepest muscle of the flexor group is the short head of the *biceps femorus,* which joins with its twin, the long head, to form a common tendon that inserts into the head of the fibula, the outer bone of the lower leg. The remaining muscles in the flexor group all arise from the ischial tuberosity. The wider semi-membranous inserts into the posterior aspect of the tibia. The thinner semi-tendinous inserts on the anterio-medial surface of the tibia. Leg-extension moves are the best exercises to build and peak the back of the thighs.

In the calf area, the larger and deeper muscle is the *soleus,* which originates from both the fibula and the tibia. The smaller *gastrocnemius* has two heads, one originating from the lateral aspect and the other from the medial of the lower femur. Both heads join to overlay the soleus and to insert into the Achilles tendon.

1. SQUATS—I've already talked about the squat with the basic exercises.

Now that you will be using heavier weights I would recommend that you not do a full squat, or sit all the way down, because according to orthopedic surgeons this could be harmful to your knees. Go three quarters of the way down, until your thighs are roughly parallel to the floor, and come back up. Keep your upper body straight. If you lean forward, you will train your lower back more than your thighs. Concentrate on the thigh muscle right now and keep your head straight up.

The squat can be done in different ways, depending upon your need and purpose. If you have problems developing the outside of your thigh, you should keep your feet parallel and close together. If you need more on the inside you should point your toes out and put your feet farther apart. You can also put a bench underneath for protection when you do the squat in case you can't come up again.

I recommend five sets of 8 repetitions, or a total of 40. Note: Always start with lighter weights and work your way up. Start with 100 pounds the first set. The next set go to 120, then 140, then 160, then 180, then

200. Move up slowly but surely. The last set ought to be so hard you can do only 5 or 6 repetitions. That is the set that should prepare you for your next workout. The first set is the warm-up set; the last should always be the power set.

2. LEG EXTENSIONS—Except for the squat, there is no better exercise for developing the whole leg. Leg extensions build the front and back thigh muscles, strengthen the knees, and stretch and tone the calves.

The machine for this exercise consists of a bench with a padded lever bar at one end. Sit at the end of the bench with your knees well back to the edge and grasp the sides of the bench slightly behind you to brace yourself. You can either hook your feet under the bar, as shown in the photos, or point them behind it. Pointed feet tend to focus the exercise on the quadriceps and knees; hooked feet give the extra benefit of a good stretch of the back of the leg.

With a smooth, steady motion, push the bar up until your legs are out straight. Hold this position for a few seconds; then lower your legs at the same controlled

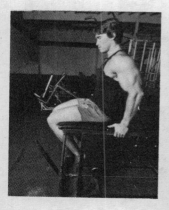
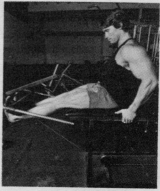

Leg extension

rate of speed, working against the resistance, and let the bar come down. You can start with 20 or 30 pounds and add weight as you progress. Work toward five sets of 12 reps.

3. LEG CURLS—We discussed this exercise thoroughly in the preceding chapter. Again, it's important to do full curls. Holding the front support firmly, you lie on your stomach and let the machine all the way down. Then bring the weight up as high as you can. Let me caution you again not to use your buttocks, lower back, or forearms to help you lift. Isolate this exercise in your leg biceps. Weight is not as important as form.

Do five sets of 8 to 10 repetitions.

Leg curl

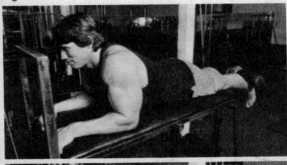

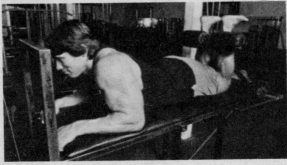

4. CALF RAISES—ON CALF MACHINE (STANDING)—We use the calf every time we walk. Each time we take a step, one calf lifts the entire body. If your body weight is 200 pounds, each step you take gives the calf a 200-pound repetition—So if you loaded the calf machine with 200 pounds, it would be roughly equal to walking. You should use more than your body weight on the machine. A lot of people don't realize that. Guys with skinny calves who weigh 200 pounds and use 150 pounds on the calf machine will still have skinny calves. The weight resistance will not help them.

In my opinion, Reg Park had the greatest calves in the world and he has trained for years with a lot of weight. As I said earlier, when I was in South Africa training with Reg I put my usual puny 150 pounds on the calf machine, and he changed it to 1000 pounds for his sets. He was doing ten sets of 10 repetitions. I realized then what it takes to get big calves. I trained with Reg and worked my way up to 500 pounds on the calf machine. My calves grew half an inch in one month. Since then I've been in the habit of training with heavy weights for my calves.

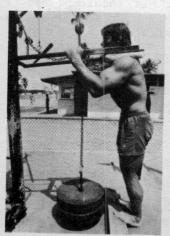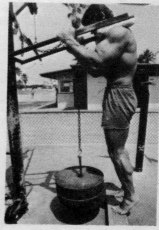

To get a perfect stretching of your calves, you should start with your toes on a high block, go all the way down to touch the floor with your heels, and then come all the way up on your toes. Only through a perfect, full movement can you develop perfect calves. A straight-on, parallel foot position is good for the all-around calf. If you want to develop the outside, point your toes in; if you want to develop the inside, point your toes out.

The calf is different from any other muscle. It is stubborn and slow to respond. You should be just as stubborn. Don't do only 8 or 10 repetitions—do at least five sets of 15 repetitions.

Chest

The muscles of the chest are the *pectoralis major, pectoralis minor, subclavius* and *serratus anterior (serratus magnus)*. The pectoralis muscles, consisting of the clavicular (upper) portion, and the sternal (lower) portion, is attached to the clavicle (collarbone), the whole length of the sternum (breastbone) and the cartilage of several ribs. The largest mass of the pectorals starts at the upper arm bone (humerus) where it fastens at a point under and just above where the deltoids attach to the humerus. The serratus fans out to cover the rib cage like armor plates.

The pectoralis muscles pull the arm across the front of the body and let you perform such actions as pitching a ball underhanded, doing a wide-grip bench press, swimming the crawl stroke, and executing parallel-bar dips. Because of their attachment to the humerus, the pectorals play an important secondary role in back exercises such as chinning. There is in fact a definite interdependence between chest and back exercises. The chest will not reach its full potential size unless the latissimus dorsi muscles are fully developed.

1. BENCH PRESS—We have discussed this exercise in a previous chapter. Concentrate on letting the weight slowly down to your chest and slowly pressing it up again. The down movement makes use of a principle called negative resistance. Which means the muscle is developed as much through controlling the down movement as through the pressing movement. So you should pay as much attention to form in letting the weight down as in lifting it up. This principle holds for almost every exercise. Do not let the weight bounce off your chest or come down only halfway. Make a full movement.

I suggest 8 repetitions, starting with a light weight and increasing it each set. Work up to a heavy weight so that you can do only 5 or 6 repetitions in the last set. This builds the basic foundation of the chest—not only the middle part of the pectoral but also the lower and upper parts.

Note: In the bench press you should keep your feet on the floor to stabilize your body.

Bench press

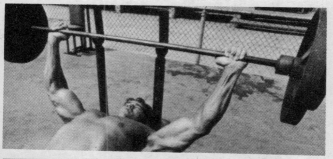

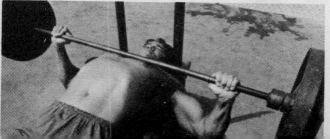

2. BENT-ARM DUMBBELL FLYES—Flyes stretch the rib cage and build the outer pectorals. They're one of my favorite exercises and have had the best effect on my pectoral muscles, causing them to grow wide and low, with a lot of definition.

Lie flat on your back on the bench. Lift your legs up and lock them in a cross position, as shown in photographs (this way you eliminate strain on your stomach). Starting with a pair of dumbbells held at arm's length over the chest, bend your arms (see photo) slightly to take the pressure off your elbows and lower the weights out to the sides as far as you can (almost to the floor) while inhaling as much air as possible. Then slowly raise your arms—exhaling and tensing the pectorals as you do—until the dumbbells are about 10 inches apart. At the top, flex your pectoral muscles and press the weight really hard.

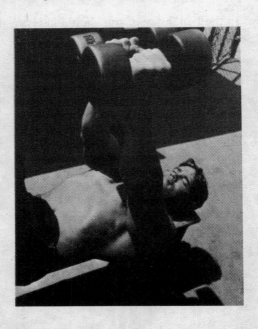

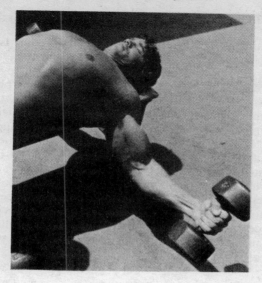

Doing a flye is like hugging a large tree. You make a wide circle with the dumbbells. A lot of guys do it with the weight so close to the pecs that it becomes a pressing movement. But you don't want a pressing movement. Another variation is to touch the dumbbells at the top, but that is not what we are after on this routine. By stopping the dumbbells about 10 inches apart, you keep a constant tension in the pectoral muscles—particularly the outer portions—which pumps them and promotes rapid growth. Be sure to get a full stretch by slowly lowering the dumbbells as far as possible on each repetition.

Do five sets of 10 repetitions.

Abdomen

I think a beautifully developed midsection is the most immediately impressive part of the male physique. If you are familiar with Greek mythology or classical sculpture you have no doubt seen the photographs of the various gods and how each had fantastic abdominal muscles. Well-sculptured, highly defined abdominals give the physique a more finished appearance than any other muscle group. In competition, if your abdominal region has a slight layer of fat on it, you might as well forget about winning a trophy.

Sharply defined abdominals are a must for maximum impressiveness. The entire abdominal region needs to be thoroughly exercised to get rid of all the visible surface fat. The following exercise routine will give your midsection sensational cuts.

1. SIT-UPS—KNEES BENT—Keep your legs locked in a bent position throughout this familiar exercise. Exhale as you sit up, inhale as you return to the starting position on the floor. If you don't have an abdominal board, or slant board, hook your feet under some heavy object such as a bed or a dresser. A towel or sponge over the feet for padding will make this more comfortable.

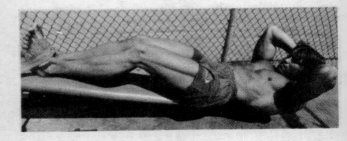

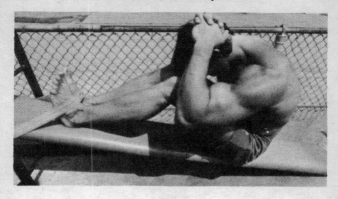

I would go to 200 repetitions a day, approximately—not all at once, but the way you feel good about it. So it can be two times 100 or six times 35.

2. LEG RAISES—KNEES BENT—Do at least 200 repetitions, or until you really feel the burn.

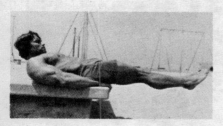

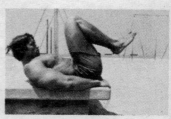

3. WRIST CURL—As I have said, you should do this exercise every day to build up your forearms. You use the forearm every day, therefore you can train it every day. Let the weight down as far as you can, and bring it up as far as you can. This is the most basic, the best, and the easiest exercise for forearms, and you can use a lot of weight.

Do at least five sets of 15 repetitions and continue the final set until it is impossible to squeeze out another fraction of an inch of wrist movement.

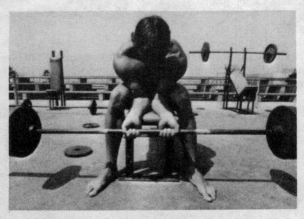

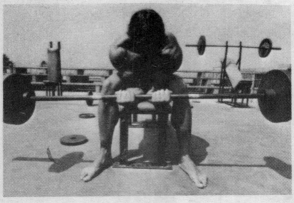

TUESDAY AND FRIDAY PROGRAM

On Tuesday and Friday you will work on shoulders, back, arms, abdominals and calves. The reason for combining these body parts is this: I believe pressing movements and pulling movements should be done together. Most shoulder work is a pressing movement and all the back exercises are pulling movements. The shoulders, the back and the arms are all connected, so it makes sense also to train the arms. By the time you finish the shoulder workout, which involves a lot of triceps movements, and the back workout, which involves a lot of biceps movements, the arms are thoroughly warmed up. You can then proceed to the arm exercises.

Shoulders

In the shoulders, both the deltoids and the trapezius should be developed equally. Add a nice V-shaped trap to a wide deltoid and you have the perfect combination for a powerful, impressive-looking back.

The *deltoidus* is a thick, large triangular muscle that covers the shoulder joint in the front, behind and laterally. It encircles the cap of the shoulder. The muscle fibers converge to unite in a thick tendon which inserts into the middle lateral side of the upper arm bone. The muscle's basic action is to lift the arm away from the body. It makes sense then that forward, lateral and backward movements are necessary to work the muscle fully.

The *trapezius* is a flat triangular muscle that covers parts of the neck, shoulders and upper back. It arises from the base of the skull, reaches out to the deltoids, runs down the nuchal ligament of the neck and then attaches to the spine in the area of the twelfth thoracic vertebra. Its function is to raise and lower the scapula and help lift the shoulders from the front. Fully developed, it creates a dramatic mass of rippling muscle between the deltoids when the arms are flexed.

1. PRESS BEHIND NECK—The press behind neck develops only the front of the deltoid. Do this exercise in a standing position. Grip the barbell just wider than your shoulders. Let the bar down until it touches behind your neck, then press the weight all the way up and lock your arms. Many people only allow the weight to drop as far as the back of their head. This is not enough. You must make the full movement, that extra 4 or 5 inches down to the neck, in order to get a complete stretch in the front deltoid.

Note: When you do any kind of pressing movement, push the weight straight up. Feel strong with the weight and don't let it overcome you.

Do five sets of approximately 8 repetitions. Start with less weight and work your way up. The last set should be 6 repetitions with a significant weight increase to insure a good pump.

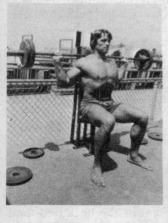
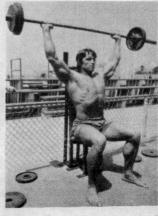

2. LATERAL RAISES—Lateral raises work specifically on the side and rear deltoid. I do this exercise in a slightly bent-over position so that there is little chance to borrow force from other muscles. Start with the dumbbells in a low position near the thighs and lift

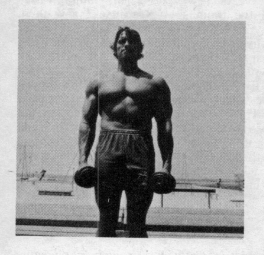

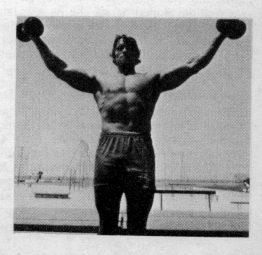

them up just higher than your shoulders. The way you control the effectiveness of the exercise is by turning the wrist. If you turn the wrist with the thumb up you will affect only the front deltoid with the pressing movement.

For many years I was doing my lateral raises wrong—with the thumbs up—because I saw them done that way in pictures, in magazines. I could never figure out why my rear deltoids didn't grow. Then once I was experimenting at home and I found that by turning the wrist to the side and making it straight, like a horizontal fist, with the thumb pointed toward the front and the weight straight, I got sore in my rear deltoid area. The more I turned the little finger up, the more the strain would go into the rear deltoid. So while I was coming up with the dumbbells I started turning my wrist as though trying to pour a pitcher of water and my rear deltoids made incredible gains.

Do approximately five sets of 8 to 10 reps.

Back

The single most dramatic feature of a great physique is a well-developed back. The back balances out the body by tying together the major muscle groups and giving the whole thing a symmetrical look. The exercises you will be doing in this section are for the three major muscle groups of the back:

The *trapezius*—which we already discussed in the section on shoulder development.

The *latissimus dorsi*—which is a large, triangular expanse of muscle that starts in the lumbar region of the back and then fans out wide at the top near the shoulders. Its function is to bring the arms to the center of the body and rotate them inward. It also draws the shoulders downward and backward. Well-developed "lats" give the dramatic V taper to the upper body and enhance just about every pose from the front and back, both relaxed and tensed.

The *spinal erectors*—consist of several muscles in the lower back region which guard the nerve channels and help keep the spine erect. These muscles should be developed to give the back a finished look.

Back development should not be thought of simply in terms of appearance. Several other muscle groups depend upon it for increases in size and strength. For instance, even if you never performed any specific exercises for the arms, they would grow bigger and stronger from heavy back work. Then too, if you ever hope for a 50-plus-inch chest, you'll never get it unless your back is fully developed—the back makes up almost half of the chest measurement.

The back is a big important area of muscles and it should be trained really hard.

1. CHIN-UPS BEHIND THE NECK—The chin-up is strictly for the latissimus, which gives you width. The pressure pulls apart your shoulder blades and stretches the lats.

Hang on the bar with a wide grip, much wider than your shoulders. Lift your body up until the bar touches

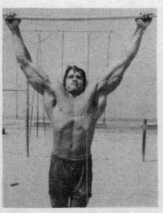
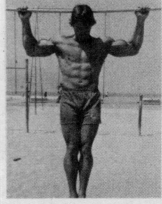

behind your neck. Let yourself down slowly. Keep
your legs slightly bent, but don't make any cheating
movements with the waist or hips. Nothing should
move except your arms.

By now you ought to be able to do 10 reps without
stopping. Do six sets, for a total of 60.

2. ROWING WITH BAR—BENT-OVER POSITION—
This is a basic exercise to widen and thicken the upper
back and add density to the lower back. Stand on an
exercise bench as I am doing in the photograph. Bend
forward at the waist so your upper back is parallel to
the floor, and grasp the barbell with a medium-wide

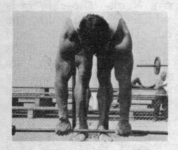

Rowing with bar—
bent-over position

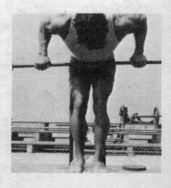

grip. Keep your knees slightly bent. Pull the bar up until it touches your stomach, then lower slowly for a full stretch of the upper back muscles. Don't allow the weight to touch the floor; keep your back in constant tension until you have completed all 12 repetitions. It is important too to make the back muscles do all the work. Don't tense the biceps as you pull upward; think of the hands and arms as hooks.

Always let the bar all the way down to your toes. That's why I prefer to do this exercise standing on a bench; on the floor, the weights will not let the bar go to my toes, and the back is not stretched completely. When you lift the bar, pull it to the waist area. If you pull it to the chest, your elbows can't move back far enough. Don't swing too much with your upper body or come up too high.

Guys who do not row never win a contest. Without doing this exercise you will not get a wide, muscle-studded back, and without a great back you can't hope to win a competition. Even if you don't compete, you need rowing to develop the vital muscles around the spine. You can get really strong by lifting. That's why I've combined chin-ups with rowing—to make the back wider and thicker.

When I met Roger Callard, Mr. Western America, he had been doing chin-ups all his life. He had a wide back, but never a winning back. He could hit a straight-on back pose in a contest and nothing happened. A year ago I encouraged him to start rowing; as a result of his efforts he now wins the Best Back in every contest. Bent-over rowing is hated by most bodybuilders because you're in a bent-over position and your lungs and your heart are squeezed together and you can't breathe well. But it's important and should not be neglected.

Do five sets of 12 repetitions.

Arms—Biceps and Triceps

To some people the biceps are the symbol of strength. Everybody can relate to arms. Arms are one of the most impressive parts of the body, the part everybody wants to see. When somebody says, "Show me your muscles," you don't show your calves. You automatically lift up your arm and flex your bicep. A lot of attention should be put into arms so they look good.

The upper arm is made up of two muscle groups— the biceps and the triceps. As the prefix "bi" implies, the bicep has two parts. The short head arises from a tendon attached to the corocoid process of the scapula and inserts into the upper portion of the radius bone of the forearm. It aids in the flexion of the upper arm, shoulder and forearm. The long head of the biceps originates from the supra glenoid tuberosity of the upper arm bone and inserts in a common tendon sheath with the short head into the forearm. Its major function is the flexion of the forearm. The tricep is composed of three muscles with a common tendonous attachment—hence the name triceps. The long head arises from a tendon on the scapula; the lateral from the posterior surface of the upper arm (humerus) bone; and the medial head has its origin in an area just below that of the lateral head. All three insert into a single tendon attached to the forearm. The action of the triceps is to extend the forearm, with the long head also aiding in bringing the arm closer to the body from a lateral position.

Biceps

1. BARBELL CURL—STANDING—Grip the bar shoulder-width, letting it rest against your thighs. Curl the bar up with only your forearms. Your upper arm should remain in the same position throughout the ex-

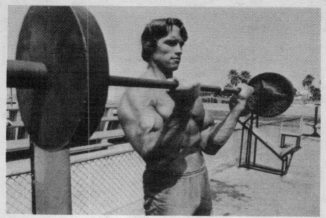

Barbell curl

ercise. It's important that you don't borrow from your other muscles. Flex your biceps firmly at the top of the curl. Lower the bar slowly and repeat.

Use the add-weight rep system for five sets of 8, 8, 6, 6, 6 reps.

2. DUMBBELL CURL—SITTING—The dumbbell curl is similar to a barbell curl except you use two dumbbells. The reason for the dumbbells is that they allow you to turn your wrist while doing the curl and reach some neglected areas of the biceps. The result is more resistance from the dumbbell curl than the standing barbell curl.

I start my dumbbell curl with my knuckles facing the front, as shown in photo. As I lift the weights, I turn them gradually until my palms are up, and then I flex the biceps. This turning of the wrist gives the biceps an extra edge they wouldn't otherwise get. Do the movements slowly and deliberately. Move only your forearms. Each time you lower the weights you should

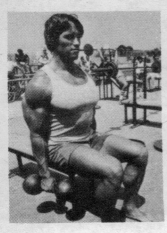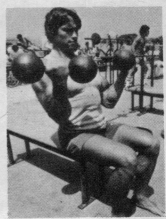

let them hang completely loose—not three-quarters of the way down.

Do five sets of 8 repetitions and do the turning each set.

3. RESTRICTED INCLINED DUMBBELL CURL—One of the world's greatest bodybuilders was Steve Reeves. Aside from his classic proportions, he had incredible arms. One of Reeves' favorite biceps exercises was the inclined curl with dumbbells. I used this exercise early in my career. But I realized I wasn't getting the same results Reeves was. I experimented and discovered a simple trick that changed the whole exercise for me. I held my elbows slightly forward and thus kept the weights from merely swinging upward as I curled. Now instead of letting the front deltoid help, I restricted the work to my biceps. The difference was unbelievable. Almost immediately I noticed a new peak to my biceps.

Assume the position slowly in the first photograph and curl the dumbbells slowly up to the finished position. Remember, if you feel your deltoid doing the

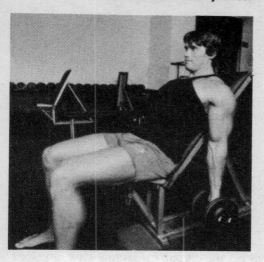

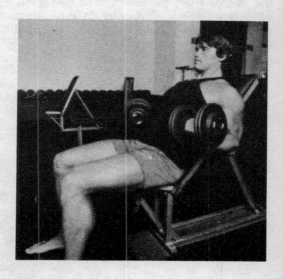

lifting you are doing it wrong. Isolate it for your biceps.

Do five sets of 10 repetitions.

Note: One thing about the biceps—you need to relax them completely between repetitions. Stand with your arms limp, and the outside of your hands turned toward the thighs. This gives the blood a chance to flow freely through the biceps.

Triceps

1. STANDING FRENCH PRESS—WEIGHT BEHIND NECK—In review, the standing French press requires a very full movement. The bar should go from being totally extended, all the way down to the back of the neck. Keep your elbows parallel, straight up and down, and move only your forearms. This develops the triceps from the elbow area all the way down to your lats. A lot of people do this exercise with a curved bar, which is acceptable, but my own preference is a classic straight bar.

Do five sets of 12 repetitions.

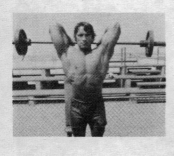
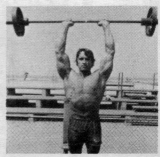

2. LYING TRICEPS EXTENSION WITH BAR—This is a direct exercise with traces the triceps all the way down from the elbow to the latissimus.

Lie down with your head hanging off the bench. Let the weight come down to the level of your forehead and press it up again. Do not press the weight above your chest. The weight should remain behind your head, as in photo. Hold your elbows slightly back and parallel. Again, let only your forearms move.

Do five sets of 10 to 12 repetitions.

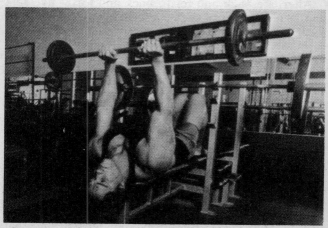

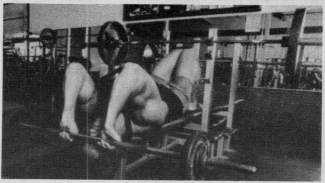

Abdomen

For your abdominals workout you should alternate
one set of leg raises with bent legs with one set of
twists with the broomstick in a bent-over position.
You combine them in order to save time. The leg
raises are for the abs, and bent-over twists are for the
obliques, at the side of the waist. Spend no more than
7 minutes on the whole program. And don't worry
about resistance. Repetition is most important in waist
training. The object is just to burn off the fat.

Alternate back and forth, back and forth, five sets
and 20 repetitions of each exercise for a total of 100 of
each.

Forearms

WRIST CURLS—Do five sets of 15 repetitions.

WEDNESDAY

Work on your weak points. After you have trained
long enough to discover your weak points, write them
down and analyze them. You should know by now if
your leg biceps aren't as fully developed as the front of
your thighs, or your latissimus isn't progressing as
well as your chest. Every bodybuilder will find that
certain parts of his body don't respond as well as
others. These areas require extra work and should be
the focus of your Wednesday workout.

When I first started training, my left bicep stayed a
half to three-quarters of an inch smaller than my right
one. It was the result of something I was doing wrong.
So I spent one day just training that one bicep with a
dumbbell. A few weeks later I had evened it out with
the right arm.

On these weak-point days, flex the muscles that are
giving you trouble, flex them continuously. Flex, pose,

and with your mind try to send a rush of blood into the muscle. With this additional attention it will slowly come up to standard.

Three-quarters of an hour ought to be sufficient for training your weak points. Do no more than six or seven sets of 10 repetitions for each body part.

A Word of Caution

By this time, a lot of people feel overconfident and want to get into a six-day-a-week routine. You should not push yourself. In fact, if you feel you have no weak points you should not put in a fifth day. Rest, let your body relax and grow. Work up gradually and don't blow it. Sometimes you can do so much your mind gets sick of it. Remember what I said earlier: Keep your mind hungry. People have a tendency to overdo things at first and then sluff off. Your should keep up this four-day routine for three months if you're going to be a competitive bodybuilder. If you're not planning to go into competition, stay with this program for six months.

Chapter Five
Accelerated Training
(Six Days a Week)

In recent years bodybuilding has made incredible advances. Bodybuilders are now bigger and better than ever. The average contest winner today is not only bigger than the competitors of the past but he has more muscularity. Modern training methods, new innovations in equipment, and improved knowledge of nutrition (including the use of modern food supplements) have enabled bodybuilders to reach the kind of perfection it takes to be a contest winner faster.

This evolution in bodybuilding is paralleled in other sports too, thanks to a new favorable assessment of weight training. Athletes today are stronger and faster than their predecessors. Weight-trained athletes consistently break world records in all sports. Many of the mythical "barriers"—such as the 70-foot shot put, the 28-foot broad jump, the 18-foot pole vault, the 500-pound standing press, the 650-pound bench press—have been exceeded through knowledge, training and confidence.

Bodybuilders today try to develop their bodies to the fullest, which means building up the muscles to their maximum possible size while retaining shape and definition. No champion bodybuilder is ever satisfied until he has reached his ultimate potential of muscle size and muscularity and then honed it down with perfect cuts. These are the things that you should be concerned with in Chapter Five.

MONDAY AND THURSDAY PROGRAM

Legs
Calves
Waist

Legs

No area in bodybuilding is more neglected than the legs. When people ask you to show your muscles, they expect you to take off your shirt and show the upper body. Of course, you want to develop what people want to see. The drive to develop the lower portion of the body isn't usually as great. Another reason many bodybuilders steer away from extensive leg work is that it's very difficult. The thighs are powerful and need great amounts of weight, and the calves are stubborn and need a lot of reps. If you're not willing to work, then you can forget about getting championship legs.

If you want to enter physique competition, you'll never win any big titles without having the balanced physique a good pair of legs gives you. In the process of getting those legs, the work will give you tremendous endurance and help add inches of muscle to almost every area of the body. Not to mention that your metabolism and the general functioning of your organs will be enhanced by the work you do for your legs.

1. SQUATS—You will hear countless arguments against the squat. Some people say it increases the size of the gluteus maximus to ridiculous proportions. Others say its only effect is to weaken the knees and lower back. These arguments are all without foundation. The squat is the best thigh-building exercise I know. At the same time, it conditions the whole cardiovascular system.

Choose a weight that makes you work for 10 repetitions. Do five sets.

2. Leg Extensions—With leg extensions, the combination of weight and strict form will work to stimulate all the muscles around the knee and separate the lower thigh. It is most important to make full repetitions, allowing the weight to drop to the bottom and then to lift it until your legs are totally straight.

Do five sets of 10 repetitions.

3. Leg Curls—By this time you will have been doing leg curls for at least a year. Be sure you have not become negligent. Many bodybuilders let their buttocks come up and assist in the curl. This takes away from its effect on the leg biceps. Pull only with your legs, drawing your heels all the way to your buttocks. If you get tired in the final reps, have your training partner help you make the full movement.

Do five sets of 12 repetitions.

4. Lunges—The lunge is an exercise most bodybuilders disregard, claiming it is archaic. However, for years I have included it with my basic exercises. I know no other exercise that is so effective in separating the entire thigh muscle.

In the beginning try a few practice lunges with a light barbell. Rest the bar behind your neck. Step forward in a lunging motion, allowing the forward foot to fall flat and the leg to bend almost 45 degrees, while the trailing leg remains straight, with the heel raised. Then, pushing with the forward leg, lift your body back to a standing position. Put power into each lunge. After a few repetitions you will feel the four heads of the quadriceps start to burn.

Form is even more important in doing lunges than it is in most exercises. To make sure you are moving ahead smoothly and keeping the bar balanced, I suggest you do this in front of a mirror.

Do five sets of 8 to 10 repetitions.

Calves

1. STANDING CALF RAISES ON A CALF MACHINE—
If you have been working seriously on your calves, you will now be doing this exercise with considerably more weight than when you began. The results of your diligence should be starting to show. You may now want to hit different areas of the calf. By pointing your toes inward you can reach the outer head of the calf; by pointing your toes outward the stress goes to the inside of the calf.

Do five sets of 15 repetitions.

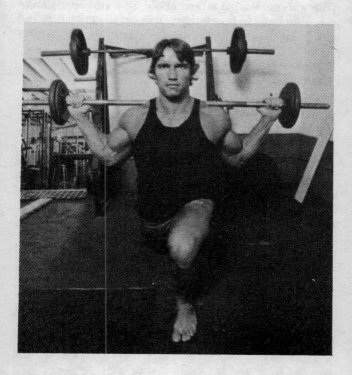

2. Sitting Calf Raises on a Calf Machine—
When you sit to perform calf raises a greater amount of
work is done by the lower part of the calf and the
soleus muscle, which runs down the outside of the shin
and connects into the heel. By placing the weight directly above your knees, you isolate the exercise
specifically to your calves.

Rest your toes on the wooden block. Work the muscle through a full range of movement. When you reach
the top, hold it and flex the calves hard; then slowly let
the calf stretch all the way down to the bottom. Keep
your torso perfectly still and do the lifting with only
your calves. We've talked about how stubborn calves
are. You have to bomb them in order to get growth. So
after you can no longer do full reps, do partial reps
until the calf literally refuses to move.

Do five sets of at least 15 repetitions.

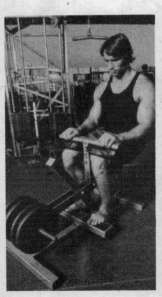 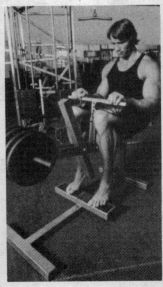

Waist

1. SIT-UPS—KNEES BENT—At this point you can easily do five sets of 50 repetitions. Each time you finish a set, pull your upper body into a knot, cramping your abs, and hold it for 20 to 30 seconds.

2. LEG RAISES—In doing this exercise, don't let your feet touch the floor. This will keep the abs under continuous tension.
Do five sets of at least 50 repetitions.

3. TWISTS—While holding an empty bar on the back of your shoulders, with your waist sucked in, exhale as you rapidly twist as far as possible, first to the right, then to the left. This really burns up any fat on the obliques.
Do five sets of 50 repetitions.

Wrist Curl

It should be automatic by now for you to go to the bench for wrist curls at the end of each day. Remember this exercise not only develops the forearm, it also increases gripping power and wrist strength.
Do five sets of 12 repetitions. If you are not having to strain out the last 3 reps you are not putting enough weight on the bar.

TUESDAY AND FRIDAY PROGRAM

Back
Chest
Shoulders

The Tuesday and Friday program is for the back, chest and shoulders. I explained in a previous chapter why you ought to follow this sequence. In my experience these three muscle groups fit together. Naturally, later on you can split them up for different reasons, but right now you should continue to work on them together.

Back

1. CHIN-UPS—I have put chin-ups first because they are a hard exercise and you should do them in the beginning, when you're strongest.

Start with regular chin-ups, doing them as you have been. Do some of the chin-ups into the back of the neck and others to the chin. Always make sure you get a variation of this exercise. I like to do a combination—one set to the front, one set to the back.

Your grip should be wide, much wider than your shoulders. Use a chinning bar with the ends bent down slightly, which gives you a different pull on your latissimus. It's a better, more direct way of doing chin-ups than using a straight bar.

Do five sets of 10 to 12 repetitions. If you are light, have a lot of pulling power, and feel 12 repetitions are easy, put some extra weight around your waist. Tie a 10- or 20-pound plate to your training belt with a string.

When you finish each set of chin-ups, do some stretching exercises on the bar. Let's say you've done 10 repetitions and couldn't do another one: try two or three half-movements, just to pull the shoulder blades apart.

2. ROWING WITH BAR—Rowing with a bar gives you thickness in the back. Stand on a bench, take a grip wider than your shoulders, and let the bar down to your toes; remain in a bent-over position and pull the bar all the way up to your waist. Your knees don't have to be locked; they can be a little loose for more support and flexibility. Do full movements. The reason for the wider grip is to make your elbows go as far

back as possible. I've found that the more the elbows move back the better it is for building your center back, which is often neglected.

Do five sets of 10 reps, using as much weight as you can handle.

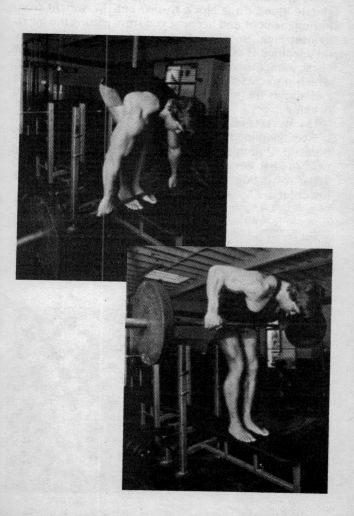

3. T-BAR ROWING—This is a new exercise which will add dramatic thickness to the outside of your lats. One end of the bar is connected to the floor, and on the other end is a short handle that will allow you to take a close grip and pull the weight up to your chest. You should stand on a block to prevent the weight from hitting the floor and keeping you from getting the maximum stretch. Because of your narrow grip and the way the machine is constructed, the plates will touch your chest sooner than the bar does in the wide-grip rowing, which prevents your elbows from moving back as far and allows the muscles in the outside of your back to develop.

Do five sets of 10 reps.

I've combined these three exercises for the back because chin-ups work on width, bent-over rowing with the bar develops the center and lower back, and T-bar rowing develops the outside of the back and the lower lats.

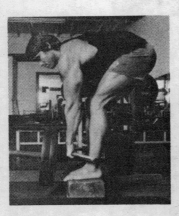

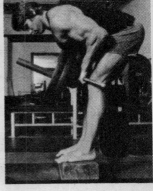

Stretching and Flexing

After your back work is completed you need to do a lot of stretching, a lot of flexing to avoid stiffness. Grasp a stationary bar and pull, bowing your back until you feel all the muscles widening and flattening. Vary your foot positions and your hand positions on the bar in order to reach every area of the back. Let yourself relax completely.

Right from the beginning, while you are developing your muscles, you should also be flexing them and working to gain control over them. Do a double biceps pose to control your back and check it in a mirror. Then try to flex each individual muscle in the back. Work on this until you have complete control over your muscles. The way to the top in competitive bodybuilding is not merely to have muscles but to be able to control your muscles and to show them. Remember that most of the points in a physique competition are achieved through posing.

Chest

1. BENCH PRESS—This is a growth-stimulating exercise I have used since I first began training. When you are at the stage you are now, it not only pumps the blood over the entire pectoral area but also increases your muscle depth.

Use a medium-wide grip, about 24 inches. Lower the bar until it touches your chest, approximately half an inch above the nipples, then ram it back to the starting position without the aid of a bounce—just use pure pectoral power. Inhale deeply as you lower the bar, and exhale as you push it up. Add weight each set. For example, on the first set I start out with a warm-up set of 12 to 15 reps. On the second set I will add weight and do 10 reps; on the third set, more weight and 8 reps; more weight and 6 reps on the fourth set; more weight and 4 to 6 reps on the fifth set.

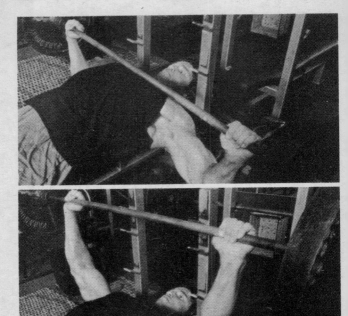

Use so much weight you can barely make the final repetitions. Add 20 or 30 or 40 pounds each set. The reason for using increasing amounts of weight is to prepare the muscle for a greater beginning weight in your next workout. You want to build power, speed and size.

I suggest doing bench presses with stands where you can catch the barbell if it becomes necessary. Or have your training partner stand behind you to help you with the last few repetitions.

2. BARBELL INCLINE PRESS—The inclined press with a barbell builds the upper pectoral, concentrating

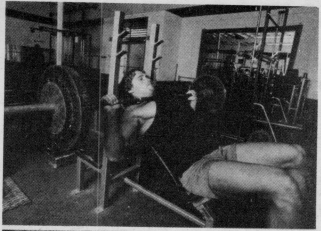

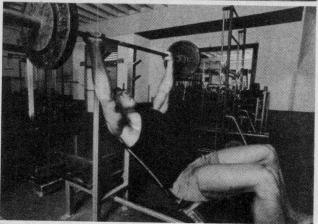

Barbell incline press

on the area where that muscle ties into the front deltoid. Although the bench press reaches a little into the upper pectoral muscle, the inclined press attacks it directly. It gives that "armor-plated" look to the upper chest and helps fill in hollow spaces around the clavicle (collarbone).

Do the inclined press on a 45-degree inclined bench, with a stand to take the weight off the arms when they are in the locked position. Watch the bar with your eyes. The bar should end up two or three inches away from your chin—not on your chest.

Hold the bar slightly wider than your shoulders, using approximately the same grip as for the bench press. Lower it smoothly down and press it up again, tensing the pectoral muscles at the top. Inhale deeply as the weight is lowered, exhale as you push it overhead.

Do five sets of 8 repetitions. Again start with a lighter weight and work up. Obviously, because of the angle, you can't use as much weight in an inclined press as in a bench press.

3. BENT-ARM FLYES—Never allow the position of the dumbbells to change while you are doing this exercise. Many people turn the dumbbells. That's wrong.

Bent-arm flyes

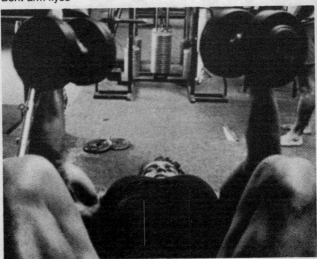

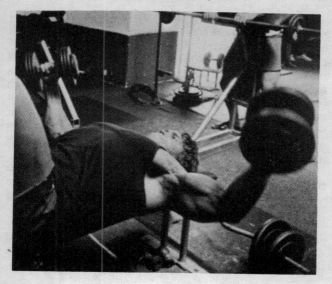

Keep them parallel at all times. Don't lift them in a pressing movement or twist your wrists. This is a total waste of time because it affects the shoulder instead of the pecs.

I consider myself a master of flying motions. I rarely see anybody using the correct form. But people I've taught to do it the right way have developed incredibly huge pecs. One of them is Franco. I taught him the flying motion in Munich in 1966. Since then he's been using 95 or 100 pounds in the strict style and he's built incredible pectoral muscles.

Do five sets of 10 to 12 repetitions.

You won't need to stretch after doing this exercise. The force of the weight going down pulls so much at the pectoral muscles in the rib cage that it is already a perfect combination of flexing and stretching.

4. PULL-OVER WITH DUMBBELL—This is the best possible movement for expanding the thorax and enlarging the rib cage. It also stretches the pectoral muscle and the latissimus, aids in developing the serratus muscles, pulls hard at your bone structure, and helps tone up the abdominals. It's a fantastic exercise which can help increase your chest measurement considerably. I have found the pullovers more effective if you lie across a flat bench rather than positioning yourself lengthwise on it. I also get a far better stretch using a dumbbell than I do with a barbell.

Pull-over with dumbbell

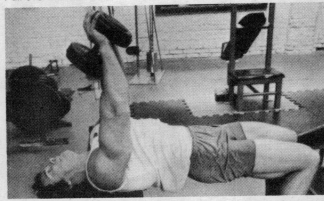

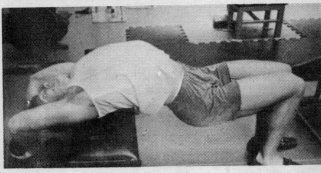

Lie across an exercise bench as I am doing in the photograph. Flatten your hands against the inside plates at one end of the dumbbell and hold it at arm's length over your chest. Only the upper back ought to be in contact with the bench. Keep your hips low throughout the exercise. Lower the dumbbell, while inhaling deeply, until it is in line with your head, then exhale as you return the weight to starting position. Inhale as deeply as possible—force all the air you can into your lungs—and keep your chest expanded—even after you exhale. In other words, keep the chest held high throughout the entire movement of this exercise.

Choose a weight that will permit you to do five sets of 15 repetitions.

Shoulders

I grouped the muscles for the Tuesday and Friday program in an unusual way, taking the back first. But this is logical. The back is a big muscle area with a lot of square inches to develop, and it should get the most attention in the beginning, when you have the most energy. Second was the chest, which is a smaller muscle group. Third are the deltoids, even smaller than the chest. The reason I put the deltoids last is not that they're unimportant. They're beautiful and complex muscles. But they are much easier to pump and develop than either the back or the chest.

1. PRESS BEHIND NECK—This exercise is an old standby. It also happens to be one of my favorites for deltoid work. Placing a barbell behind my neck, I take a medium-wide grip and then press the weight overhead. The ideal way is to do it on a bench which has a board to support the back, and then to do full movements, letting the weight all the way down and pressing it all the way back up again. Keep the bar straight.

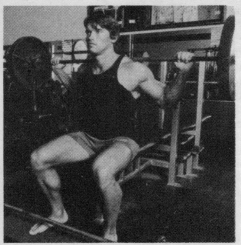

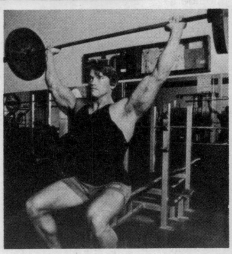

Presses behind the neck should be done in front of a mirror so you can correct yourself. Press the bar evenly.

Do five sets of 10 to 12 reps.

2. LATERAL RAISES—Lateral raises work on the side deltoid muscle. I described this exercise before. But then you were doing the rear deltoids. Now you should concentrate on the side deltoid. You only need to turn the dumbbell slightly—just enough to keep it straight. Do this exercise in a slightly bent-over position so that there is no chance to cheat. With a dumbbell in each hand, raise the weights to shoulder height and then lower them slowly. The weight must start from a dead stop, so that there is little or no swing.

Do five sets of 8 repetitions.

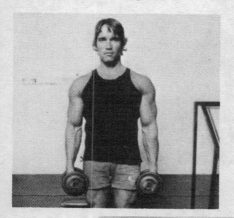

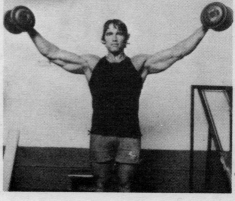

3. LATERAL RAISES IN BENT-OVER POSITION—The bent-over lateral raises are strictly for the rear deltoids. In an advanced program you need to work toward developing every area of each muscle. The rear deltoid is usually neglected, but it can be reached when you are in a bent-over position.

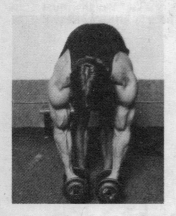

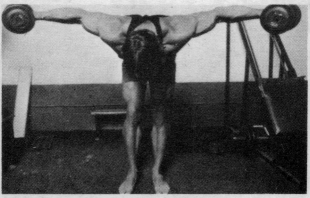

Hold your upper body parallel to the floor with the weights together in front of your legs and lift the weights toward the outside. Your palms should be facing your body. Raise the dumbbells smoothly and evenly and as high as you can to really feel the effect in your rear deltoids.

As with presses behind the neck and lateral raises, choose a weight you can handle in perfect form and do five sets of 8 repetitions.

Wrist Curls

Concentrate on your forearms. Watch them. Try to remember how they were in the beginning. The progress you see should give you the incentive to add a couple of reps on your final set and really pump the blood in there.

Do five sets of 10 to 15 repetitions.

The Tuesday and Friday routine is a tough one. You have three major muscle groups to work on, and that's the reason I'm not suggesting any waist or calf training. Those two days of the week you can just let the waist and calves rest.

WEDNESDAY AND SATURDAY PROGRAM

Arms
Triceps
Biceps

On Wednesday and Saturday you will work on triceps, biceps, calves, waist and forearms.

In my own workouts for the upper arm, I always train the triceps first because the muscle has three heads and naturally requires the most work.

Triceps

1. TRICEPS PULL-DOWN ON MACHINE—The first triceps exercise is the triceps pull-down on the machine you usually use to do lat work. This exercise acts directly on the entire triceps, and it has numerous variations. Simply by changing the spacing of the hands or the angle of the body you can have a completely different exercise.

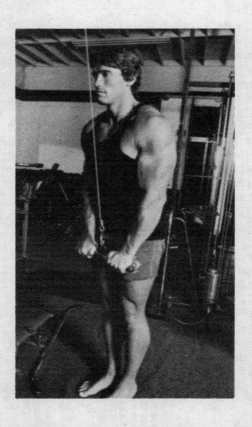

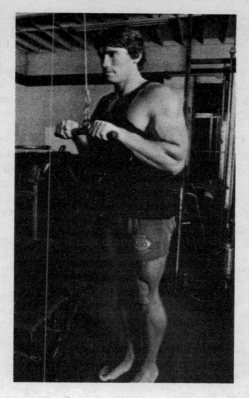

Use a bar that is bent down slightly on each side. Grip the bar with about five inches between your hands. Start with the bar right below your pectoral muscles. Then push it down until it touches your thighs. Nothing should move in this exercise except your forearms. Your pecs, your upper body, your legs and your upper arms should remain absolutely still. Force the bar all the way down with your forearms until you feel your triceps flex. You should flex the triceps on each repetition, and then let them stretch as the weight brings them up. The pulldown is an isolated exercise that builds the higher triceps near the rear deltoid area if you do it properly.

First try a warm-up set of 20 repetitions with very light weight. Then put on a heavier weight you can handle for three sets of 10 repetitions. Then add more weight and do two sets of 8 repetitions.

2. TRICEPS EXTENSION WITH DUMBBELL BEHIND NECK—The triceps extension with dumbbell behind the neck develops the entire tricep from the elbows to the shoulders. Take a light dumbbell, something you can handle for 10 repetitions, five sets, and lift the weight straight over your head, holding your upper arm against the side of your head, then let the weight slowly down behind your neck and press it up again. Only your forearm should move. The upper arm ought to remain against the side of your head and not move at all. A lot of guys turn this into a pressing movement. This is wrong. Watch yourself in a mirror. Every time your arm leaves your head you are making a mistake.

Do five sets of 12 repetitions.

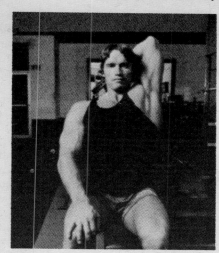

Triceps extension with dumbbell behind neck

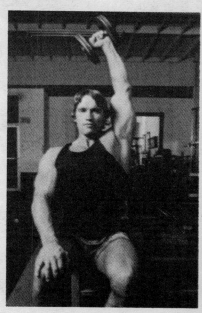

3. TRICEPS EXERCISE WITH DUMBBELLS—LYING
DOWN—The third exercise for this muscle is almost
like the barbell extension. You lie on a bench with two
dumbbells held above your face, and let them down
slowly as though you were hiding your face behind the
dumbbells. Allow nothing to move except your
forearms. Be extremely careful not to let the dumbbells down too fast, to avoid getting hit in the face.
Then press them up again slowly. The reason for using

Triceps exercise with dumbbells—lying down

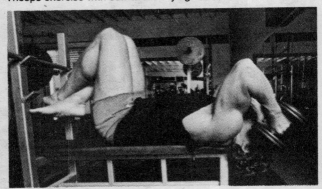

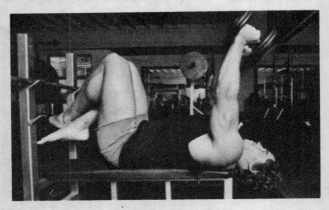

dumbbells is to allow for different hand positions. Changing the hand position changes the effect on the triceps. Experiment as you work out. You'll be able to tell the difference.

Do five sets of 8 to 10 repetitions.

Biceps

1. DUMBBELL CURL ON INCLINE BENCH—This was always one of my favorite exercises. It stretches the biceps and allows them to grow. In Austria, when I was doing the regular dumbbell curl sitting down, I felt my biceps didn't get as much stretch as they needed. So I experimented with different positions by leaning back against the wall. I discovered that this allowed my arm to swing back farther and gave more stretch to the bicep. S-T-R-E-T-C-H is what is needed in the bicep. The longer the bicep is from the shoulder to the elbow, the more it can roll up and flex and get bigger.

The dumbbell curl on an inclined bench should be done at a 45-degree angle. Start with the backs of your hands forward and slowly turn them to the outside as you pass through the middle position. When you reach

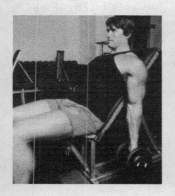
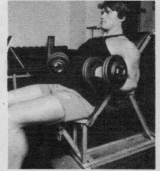

the top the backs of your hands should be toward the front again. Throughout this movement your upper arm should not change at all. Move only the forearm. If your upper arm does move, you are working your deltoid. Again, I want to stress the value of strict form. I have isolated my biceps so much that no other muscle ever gets anything out of my biceps work. Some guys say to me, "Arnold, you only use fifty-five pounds on the biceps curl—I use seventy." And it's true, they do use 70 pounds, but they have no arms. They're just worried about getting the weight up there, about ego satisfaction, and not doing the movements correctly.

Remember to turn your wrist, stretch your biceps and flex them when you reach the top position.

Do five sets of 10 to 12 repetitions.

2. PREACHER BENCH CURL—The Preacher bench curl works to increase the length of the lower part of the biceps. Grip the barbell shoulder width and lay your upper arms against the bench. Let the forearm go down slowly, then curl it back up. The movement of the bar should be slow. Let it all the way down until you feel a stretch. Halfway movements rob you of the full benefit of this exercise. When you bring the barbell up don't let the weight fall into your biceps. Flex the biceps. When you can't do any more full reps, do half- or quarter-repetitions on the top to get the top of the bicep. These are called *burns*.

Do five sets of 8 repetitions—plus the burns.

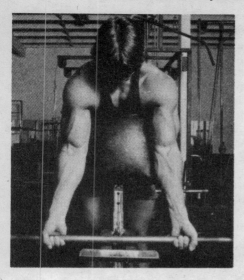

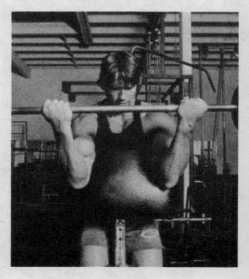

3. CONCENTRATION CURL WITH DUMBBELL—I use the concentration curl last because it is an exercise for peaking out the bicep. If you do this exercise correctly, you ought to be able to add at least a half-inch to your biceps in a few months. I use 65 pounds for this exercise, and try to do it in a strict form. Assume the position shown in the photograph, with your body bent over, one arm holding the dumbbell and the other arm braced against your knee to support your upper body. The dumbbell should be curled up to the front deltoid without moving the upper arm at all. Pull the weight slowly up to the shoulder area. It is very important not to hit the pectoral muscles with the dumbbell. This is not a rowing motion. The elbow and upper arm should

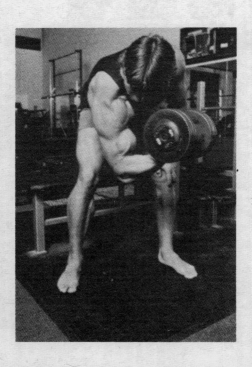

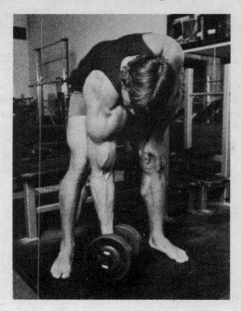

never move at all. The only movement is with the forearm. You simply lift the dumbbell to the front deltoid. Almost everyone I explain the concentration curl to does it wrong. They attempt too much weight and end up doing rowing motions with one arm, or hitting their chest with the dumbbell and not doing a full movement. Remember: Choose a weight you can handle and bring it slowly up to the front deltoid. If you do this correctly, you will get a good peak to your biceps, a bulging look.

Do five sets of 10 repetitions.

Do some stretching movements to let the blood flow through your biceps. Put your arms on the outside of your thighs and stretch the biceps.

Also, it is important after biceps and triceps training to flex both muscles forcefully.

Calves

Standing Calf Raises
Sitting Calf Raises

Go through the same routine you did for the Monday-Thursday program. Do five sets of 15 repetitions for each exercise. In addition, do a few partial reps on the final sets.

Waist

Sit-ups
Leg Raises
Twists

For your waist training, do sit-ups, leg raises and twists in exactly the same way you did Monday-Thursday. In the next chapter you'll be doing them differently.

Do five sets of 50 repetitions of each exercise.

Forearms

WRIST CURL—Do five sets of 12 repetitions. On the final rep allow the bar to remain cradled in your open fingers for as long as you can stand it, to stretch the muscles and force in more blood.

Pacing

Let's talk a little bit about time. These exercises should be done fairly rapidly. Although you are working with single sets and not supersets, you should not give yourself more than 30 to 45 seconds of rest between each set. You want to get a pump and make the muscles grow. If you don't tear down muscle tissue, you don't rebuild it, and your muscles don't grow. The only way you can get a pump is by going through your workout at a fast pace. I don't mean to do the individual exercises fast, but to move from one set to the next without undue delay. If you sit around for two minutes after each set and wait until your body relaxes, you'll never get the tight, full feeling of the pumped-up muscle. It's better to handle less weight and move fast than to handle more weight and exhaust yourself.

The entire workout in the accelerated program should not take longer than an hour and a half. If you spend more time than that on any of the routines I've outlined, you're doing something wrong.

Chapter Six
The Superset Program
(Six-Day Schedule)

When I started bodybuilding in Austria, I did only single sets. I had learned no other method of working out. I did a set, rested a minute, did another set, rested, and did another set. Then I'd change exercises and keep training the same muscle. That was it. In fact, I did single sets until I moved to Germany and started working out with some advanced bodybuilders. One of them, I remember, was Reinhart Smolana, who was already Mr. Europe and had won his height class in Mr. Universe. Another was Poldi Mercl, who had also won Mr. Universe in his height class. I noticed they were training differently. I saw them going rapidly from one piece of equipment to the next, and I wondered why they felt they needed to hurry. I thought perhaps they weren't concentrating on the exercises. I asked them about it. They explained that it was to save time. They told me there was no reason to train six hours a day, that you can do the same amount of work in three hours or four hours. I started training with them, going through this routine, combining certain exercises, cutting out rest periods. And I got incredible pumps. It was a fantastic feeling to experience a pump in the biceps and triceps or in the pecs and the lats at the same time. The pump, the combined pump, came about because we were supersetting those muscles and tying them together.

When a lot of bodybuilders pose, you can see they have great pecs, great calves and great thighs, but their bodies don't flow together. It's because they've never stopped training their muscles individually. In supersets the pump connects the muscles you are combining. Your body becomes a unit; it flows and comes together. With the combined pump, the muscles tying together, you create a need for more oxygen in your bloodstream; and when your body adjusts to that your energy level will go up, and your heart and your cardiovascular system will work better.

At this point you should have been training for at least a year. You ought to be sufficiently built up to endure a more rigorous training schedule. This is called the superset program. Supersets require an energy level high enough to allow you to go instantly from one set to the next. If you have done your foundation training faithfully, your heart and lungs should be able to handle it. What you will be doing is building your body to its ultimate size and training it for maximum definition. You will encounter mostly exercises you've been doing all along; however, you will now put them together, superset them.

There is no reason not to superset if you're in good shape. You can do more exercises in a shorter period of time, and you can get into opposite movements—pushing and pulling. You will train faster and become more accomplished. You will train muscles that are logically connected with each other or muscles on opposite sides of your body—such as the front thigh and the back thigh. Supersets will give you the feeling of progress. You'll get a double pump. You'll begin to really appreciate the condition of your body. You'll want to take it further. Having come this far, you are no longer just staying in shape, you are now changing the form of your body.

MONDAY AND THURSDAY PROGRAM

Thighs
Calves
Waist

1. SQUATS AND LEG CURLS—By supersetting the squat with the leg curl, you will be continually pumping the entire leg. Begin with the heaviest exercise, the squat, and do a warm-up set; move immediately to the leg curl machine for 10 light reps. Rest for about a minute, or long enough to let your heart slow down. However, you should not allow yourself to relax.

Repeat this cycle—squats and leg curls—for five sets, 10 repetitions per exercise per set.

2. LEG EXTENSIONS AND LUNGES—This superset will get to every muscle in your legs. Both extensions and lunges are superb for the lower thigh and the area around the knee. Lunges work the leg biceps in both the stretch and flex positions, and they warm up the calves. As I've indicated before, the effectiveness of these exercises depends largely on form. Be sure you make full repetitions.

Begin with the extensions; they will prepare your knees for the stress that lunges will put on them. Go directly to lunges. You should only rest between supersets. While you are resting, stand in front of a mirror and flex your thigh muscles. You ought to feel a deep burning sensation in the lower thighs.

Do ten supersets, 15 repetitions of each exercise.

3. STANDING CALF RAISES AND SIT-UPS—The theory behind a superset program is to save time, therefore I have combined calf raises with sit-ups. Calf raises isolate the calf muscles and take very little from the rest of the body. You can go directly from the calf machine to the bench and do 30 to 50 bent-leg sit-ups while resting your calves. Then, without a break, return to the calf machine.

Do five supersets of 15 repetitions of each exercise with no rest periods.

4. LEG RAISES AND SITTING CALF RAISES—This superset is similar to the last one. Combine your sitting calf raises with another waist exercise, the leg raises. Load the calf machine with weight and do a set of calf raises. Move directly to a bench and do leg raises with bent legs. Return, without a rest, to the calf machine.

Do five supersets of 15 repetitions of each exercise.

5. TWISTS—Do your twists in one continuous set of 50 to 100 repetitions. Assuming a bent-over position, concentrate on turning your waist in a complete half-circle and really squeezing off the inches. Then move without stopping to wrist curls.

6. WRIST CURLS—Take a weight you can handle for about 15 full reps. Then push yourself with some partial reps, even if you are able to move the bar only an inch.

Do five sets of 15 repetitions and include a few burns at the end of each set.

TUESDAY AND FRIDAY

Back and Chest
Shoulders

1. BENCH PRESS AND CHIN-UPS—Most of the upper body strength is in the chest and back, and no superset hits both these body parts as thoroughly as the bench press combined with chin-ups. After using this superset for a few weeks you will find your power in the bench press has increased considerably.

Begin with the bench press and go immediately to the bar for a few reps of chins. At the conclusion of your chins let your body hang and stretch. This pulls at the lats and pecs at the same time. Rest for a short time and return to the bench.

Do five sets of 15 repetitions for each exercise.

2. BARBELL INCLINE PRESS AND WIDE-GRIP BARBELL ROWING—A variation of the previous superset, another push-pull combination that keeps the torso completely pumped. The incline press is the paramount movement for developing the upper pectoral muscle, and rowing adds thickness to the back. In this superset it is imperative to move from one exercise to the other without rest. Pause only after a superset has been completed.

Do five sets of 12 to 15 repetitions for each exercise.

3. DUMBBELL FLYES AND T-BAR ROWING—With this combination you will hit different areas of the chest and back. The flyes provide a stretching in the pectorals necessary to counteract the constant flexing they get from the bench press. T-Bar Rowing works the inner portion of the back which is close to the spine. I attribute much of my upper back detailing to T-Bar rowing. I can't think of a much more satisfying feeling than to have the pecs and the back pumped at the same time. This superset, done without pause, will give you that double pump.

Do five sets of 10 to 12 repetitions of each exercise.

4. PULL-OVERS—A pull-over is already a combination of movements. There is no other exercise that works as directly on the rib cage, the intercostals, and the serratus muscles. It gives you additional lung capacity and increases the height of your chest carriage. If you do it with your arms fairly straight you will feel not only a stretching in the pectorals but also a pump in the latissimus.

Do five sets of 15 repetitions with very little rest between sets.

5. PRESS BEHIND NECK AND LATERAL RAISES—It may appear strange to be putting together two deltoid exercises, but there is a good reason. The press behind the neck develops the front deltoid and the lateral raises develop the side deltoid. You are training one muscle, but it is divided into three parts and these exercises isolate two of those parts.

Do five sets of 12 to 15 repetitions of each exercise.

6. BENT-OVER LATERAL RAISES AND WRIST CURLS—The reason I combine these two movements is that the bent-over lateral raise is an exercise that takes a lot of concentration to maintain the proper style, while the wrist curl is a relatively easy movement that you can do to fill the time gap between sets. Doing lateral raises in a bent-over position often calls for lighter weights; as a result, many bodybuilders tend to become sloppy in their movements. Concentrate on form. Keep your thumbs pointing down and lift the dumbbells slightly to the front. Proceed to the wrist curl without a rest.

Do five sets of 15 repetitions of each exercise.

7. CALF RAISES AND SIT-UPS—Finish the day with a vigorous workout for your calves and waist. Do a total of five sets of 15 repetitions on the standing calf raise machine. After each of these sets, go immediately to the slant board and do 50 bent-leg sit-ups.

WEDNESDAY AND SATURDAY PROGRAM

Arms

The Wednesday and Saturday routine concentrates on one area, the arms. I have divided the arm into three parts—the biceps, the triceps and the forearms.

1. TRICEPS PULL-DOWN ON MACHINE AND DUMB-BELL CURL ON INCLINE BENCH—The triceps pull-

down works on the upper part of the triceps. The dumbbell curl on the incline bench builds thickness in the biceps.

Begin with triceps pull-downs on the lat machine, using a light weight. As soon as you finish that set, pick up two dumbbells, sit on an incline bench, and do dumbbell curls for the biceps. When the superset is completed you can rest briefly. Remember, with arm work you must do full movements and get all the stretch you can.

Do five sets of 10 to 12 repetitions for each exercise.

2. TRICEPS EXTENSION WITH DUMBBELL BEHIND NECK AND PREACHER BENCH CURL—The triceps extension with the dumbbell behind your neck gets to the whole triceps, from the elbow up. The Preacher bench curl stretches the biceps and gives them more length and flexibility.

Work on your triceps first because that's the biggest and most important muscle in the arm. Do not let your upper arm move away from the side of your head. The Preacher bench curl should be done at a 75-degree slant. Doing it this way gives you more pressure in the lower biceps when the weight is down. Do not rest between sets. After you've completed a superset you can take 45 seconds. By then you should be feeling a good pump in both triceps and biceps.

Do five sets of 15 repetitions of each exercise.

3. TRICEPS PRESS LYING DOWN WITH BAR AND CONCENTRATION CURL—The triceps press lying down with the bar warms up the entire triceps, but it is more for the lower part of the muscle in the elbow area and the outside triceps. The concentration curl in the bent-over position brings peak and finish to the bicep.

Do five sets of 15 repetitions of each exercise.

4. REVERSE CURL AND WRIST CURL—The reverse curl and wrist curl are forearm exercises. The reverse

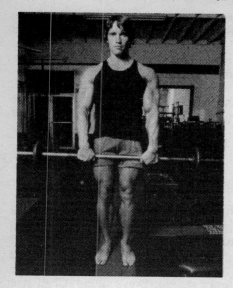

Reverse curl

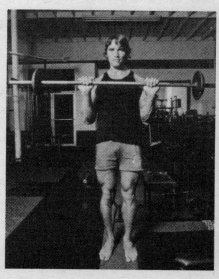

curl cuts and defines the outside and the top of the forearm, and the wrist curl builds the inside of the forearm.

The reverse curl is a new exercise. It is similar to the barbell curl except you do it with a reverse grip: refer to the photograph. Start your superset with it. Then move to the bench and do wrist curls. Burn in the last 2 or 3 reps. Take only a brief rest between supersets and stand with your hands hanging open.

Do five sets of 15 repetitions of each exercise.

Calves and Waist

On Wednesday and Saturday you should accelerate your calf and waist training. I would combine standing calf raises with bent-leg sit-ups for one superset, and alternate that with a superset of sitting calf raises and bent leg raises. Remember, to really explode the calves it takes a lot of weight. Don't skimp. Challenge yourself.

Do five sets of 15 reps of each of the four exercises.

Some Words of Advice

Do not decrease weight in any exercise. In the beginning you might feel tired as you move from bench press to chin-ups, and maybe you can only do 6 or 7 chin-ups. But that's no reason to change the weight on the bench press. Keep the weights up and try to increase your number of repetitions in the chin-ups. Push yourself. Supersetting is a tough program, but in a month or so you will adjust to it.

It's important for you to go *instantly* to the second exercise after you've finished the first one. Then at the conclusion of each superset you can rest 45 seconds to a minute. No longer. Otherwise you won't get the full benefit from supersetting. Not resting between sets also saves time, and this has a positive effect on your mind. Allow yourself an hour and 15 minutes for each workout. That is a total of 50 sets in 75 minutes. When you've done that much, you know you're getting stronger. If you can't finish your workout within this time you should punish yourself by leaving the gym. I did that in the beginning. I saw that I could handle 50 sets in an hour and 15 minutes. The next week there was a day when the hour and 15 minutes had passed and I still had 10 sets left. So I split. The whole next day I was so pissed off I'd missed doing my wrist curls and my waist that my body felt punished. From then on I got the entire program completed on time.

Importance of Positive Mental Attitude

You must approach all of your training with a positive mental attitude and the firm conviction that you will succeed. This is especially true of the superset program. Visualize the body you want and then train relentlessly until you get it. Be explicit. See yourself with that body, cut up and toned to an ideal state. Tell yourself it's possible. Then work to make it happen.

Mentally, supersetting puts an additional strain on you. Suddenly you have to focus your mind on two muscles—visualize two muscles—visualizing, for instance, how you want to pump the back and pump the pectoral muscles at the same time. You have to set your goals differently than before. The way you think and feel about your body and the way you put your mind into your muscles is entirely different now. You have to split up your attention. Sooner or later you will get used to it; you'll see the logic in making a single unit of two muscles. Gradually you will be able to go a step further and think of your whole body as a single unit over which you have complete control.

AFTERWORD

I have set down in this book a program I know from my own experience will provide you with everything you need to develop your body to its fullest potential. The process of bodybuilding does not, in my estimation, stop with the body. Seeing tremendous growth and change in yourself can open new worlds for you. Plato wrote that man should strive for a balance between the mind and the body. There should be a harmony between the two. Without a well-conditioned body, Plato felt, the mind would certainly suffer. Having worked as a bodybuilder for most of my life, I believe I have been able to create that balance within myself. I know that building the body does make the mind reach out. Strength and confidence, plus a firsthand knowledge of the rewards of hard work and persistence, can help you attain a new and better life.

Yours in good health,

Arnold